CHRONIC PAIN RELIEF

Find Relief From Your Pain With Simple
Stretching Exercises to Healing, Correct
Your Incorrect Posture and Not Allow Your
Acute Pain to Become Chronic

WILLIAM M WITTMAN

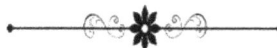

© COPYRIGHT 2020
by(William M Wittman)
All rights reserved

is without an agreement or on the other hand, any assurance affirmation.

The trademarks that are utilized are with no consent, and the production of the trademark is without authorization or support by the trademark proprietor. All trademarks and brands inside this book are for explaining purposes and are claimed by the proprietors themselves, not subsidiary with this report

DISCLAIMER

All intellect contained in this Book is given for Enlightening and informative purposes as it were. The creator isn't in any capacity responsible for any outcomes or on the other hand, results that exude from utilizing this material.

Important endeavors have been made to give data that is both precise and successful, yet the creator isn't destined for the precision or use/abuse of this data.

FOREWARD

To start with, I will jump at the chance to thank you for venturing out of confiding in me and choosing to buy/read this Life-changing eBook. Thanks for spending your time and resources on this material. I can assure you of exact results if you will diligently follow the precise blueprint, I lay bare in the information manual you are currently reading. It has transformed lives, and I firmly believe it will equally change your own life too. All the information I presented in this Do It yourself the piece is easy to digest and practice.

Table of Contents

INTRODUCTION

Everybody will encounter pain sooner or later in their lives. Pain is a fundamental type of insurance against wounds, maladies, or conditions that would some way or another weaken or even murder us. Pain alarms us that something isn't right. Pain can be either 'intense' or 'chronic' - the distinctive trademark between the two is their length.

Intense pain as a rule happens after a particular physical issue. It shows up rapidly and is normally extremely serious - one model is the pain of a messed up bone. It dies down decently fast, especially after treatment. Chronic pain, then again, appears to develop after some time, and frequently can't be associated with a specific physical issue or condition. What chronic pain keeps going in power, it compensates for in term - now and again persevering for a considerable length of time. Living with consistent pain can be horrendous, and numerous types of treatment endeavor to offer sufferers a chronic pain relief.

One of the most usually recommended treatment for chronic pain is drug, both remedy and over-the-counter. While regularly successful in mitigating pain, these are shunned by some as a result of their unfriendly reactions, which incorporate queasiness, tipsiness, and exhaustion. Others are looking for a progressively common type of chronic pain relief.

Exercise, extending and non-intrusive treatment diminish chronic joint pain and muscle irritation and fits by expanding quality, tone, and adaptability. Exercise builds blood stream, facilitates joint solidness, helps in weight reduction, and balances the pressure, uneasiness, and misery that regularly originate from living with chronic pain.

Chiropractic, needle therapy and back rub offer three elective strategies for chronic pain relief. In spite of the fact that their strategies vary, these have helped sufferers oversee chronic pain.

In the previous barely any years, analysts have started to turn their attention on the genuine wellspring of pain - the mind. Albeit a physical issue or wound may lie somewhere else on the body, signs of pain are blocked, prepared, and actually 'felt' by the cerebrum. Research discoveries demonstrate that a multidisciplinary way to deal with treating chronic pain - one that joins mental just as exercise based recuperation - gives the most chronic pain relief. Yoga, reflection, and in any event, snickering facilities have demonstrated viable medications.

The quantity of individuals experiencing spinal related pain is disturbing. Some might be enduring because of chronic pain, while others endure out of nowhere quickly following a mishap. Those looking for help with the chronic pain relief have a few choices accessible, paying little mind to the wellspring of the spinal injury. There exists a wide scope of techniques for spinal recuperating offered for those frantically looking for treatment.

The most widely recognized strategy for spinal recuperating includes a visit to a chiropractor. A chiropractor is an expert who considers the to be as a self mending life form. Normally a chiropractor will rehearse a method known as a change or spinal control.

Alterations are frequently regulated by a chiropractor when the patient is experiencing subluxation. Subluxation is when there exists a minor misalignment in the spinal vertebrae. The negative impact of subluxation is that the misalignment at last causes an unnatural measure of weight on spinal nerves.

The prosperity of the spine just as the encompassing nerves is the focal point of the network spinal analysis technique for mending. Network Spinal Analysis is regularly alluded to as the Network Chiropractic Care technique for spinal mending. This all encompassing technique towards accomplishing spinal treatment is one of the most current developments in the field of chiropractic rehearses.

Network Spinal Analysis is frequently rehearsed in focuses of wellbeing rhythms where the stream and rhythms of nerve vitality are convinced towards a characteristic state. The cozy connection between the spinal vertebrae and encompassing spinal nerves is shockingly mutually dependent. At the point when irregular weights or strain development happens in the vertebrae, at that point the encompassing nerves endure blockages and one's well-being decays.

Strategies for spinal mending are not constrained to a straightforward visit to a specialist for a painkiller remedy. Spinal mending is conceivable through a progressively comprehensive methodology that is found in the workplace of chiropractors around the globe. The benefits of such techniques as the network chiropractic care are the combination of different strategies, for example, yoga, contemplation, exercise, and different wellsprings of building individual enthusiastic quality.

It isn't uncommon to find that those needing spinal mending ought to likewise think about different techniques for self recuperating. The body is a life form that requires in general support including both the enthusiastic and physical condition. The most beneficial techniques for spinal recuperating incorporate generally speaking self mending and arrival of blocked vitality stream. Network chiropractic care is presumably one of the most advantageous techniques to accomplish total spinal mending.

Chronic pain can end up being awful understanding for the individuals who are suffering it. Be that as it may, one doesn't require to live with this condition any more. Luckily, there are meds for beating chronic pain. These medications may have certain symptoms. Be that as it may, in the event that you connect with an accomplished human service professional, you can get the most ideal drugs that would suit your clinical or wellbeing condition. Tune in to your PCP drug specialist cautiously before settling on a specific medicine. This will help you in avoiding any genuine reactions that come about because of taking these prescriptions

Here are sure compelling drugs generally recommended for treating chronic pain:

a) Acetaminophen

The medication treats chronic pain. The brand name for this drug is Tylenol. You ought to recollect that most over-the-counter and remedy pain drugs contain great measure of acetaminophen in them. Consequently, you should be extra cautious when taking pain relief meds for chronic pain.

Overdose of acetaminophen can bring about liver harm. On the off chance that, you are taking in excess of 2 acetaminophen pills daily, you have to tell your PCP.

b) Non steroidal anti-inflammatory drugs
These drugs are said to be extremely compelling in treating chronic pain. These prescriptions can be taken when you want to. At the point when taken routinely these prescriptions will in general incorporate up with blood and afterward battle the pain caused because of aggravation or expanding.

Certain meds are additionally accessible in low-portion and can be taken with no solution. In the event that your primary care physician recommends you to take non-steroidal anti-inflammatory drug, ensure that you take these with milk or nourishment. This will control the reactions identified with stomach. Taking other pain relief prescriptions related to NSAIDs is an outright no-no. On the off chance that, you need to take an alternate pain executioner, you ought to counsel your primary care physician.
c) Narcotics

These diminish chronic pain. Be that as it may, these can be addictive. Thus, you should counsel your family specialist preceding taking them. Opiates are the best choice for individuals who are experiencing serious chronic pain. These drugs should be a basic piece of their treatment. Ensure that you enlighten your PCP concerning any sort of burden you experience when taking this medication. These specialists likewise cause clogging or trouble in having solid discharges.
On the off chance that, you are on opiates you should drink in any event six to eight glasses of water regularly. Additionally eat 3 to 5 serving of vegetables and 2 to 4 serving of new organic products every day. Illuminate your PCP about blockage. The person may furnish you with certain purgatives to treat it.
d) Anti-depressants
Tricyclic anti-depressants or Duluxetine can be used to treat chronic pain.
e) Capsaicin
It is a normally possess substance found in bean stew pepper. It is used to make certain topical pain relieving creams. This drug

changes the pain flags in the skin. It squares pain without block-
ing other sensation. This medication will likewise cause a consuming sensation when previously applied. You have to wear
gloves when applying this medication.

Chronic pain is probably the best test confronting human services
experts. Customary doctors are instructed to use drugs to help
ease the indications, however become disappointed when the
drugs have inadmissible reactions which keep the patient from
playing out their ordinary day by day schedules not to mention
following a useful occupation. Non-conventional healers use of
different types of vitality medication, for example, needle therapy,
Reiki, Chinese herbs, and different common biologics are likewise
disappointed at the difficulty in finding the proper mix of treatments that have enduring impact on controlling the degree of
pain. A comprehension of the manner by which we become mindful of real sensations permits the trance inducer an exceptional
chance to keep the pain sensations from arriving at cognizant
mindfulness.

Chronic pain is by definition an impression that gives the sufferer
no useful data. Intense pain acts to caution that there is something causing harm to the body, and offers the beneficiary the
chance to make a move to stop the harm, or if nothing else get
some clinical consideration regarding manage the harm. Chronic
pain is fairly similar to a memory that won't leave. The harm has
been done, the sufferer knows as a rule of the cause for the pain,
or has discovered that there are no accessible treatments to manage the wellspring of the pain, so they keep languishing.

Every real side effect arrive at the piece of the cerebrum answerable for cognizant mindfulness by going through a structure called
the Reticular Activating System. This framework carries on rather
like a railroad exchanging framework in which the administrator
moves moving stock onto different rails, some of which permit
the train to proceed to its goal, and others are occupied to shorter
courses and are kept their anticipating stacking or emptying.
Under trance, the oblivious part answerable for controlling the reticular initiating framework is told to close down or square the
entry of chronic pain signals from arriving at cognizance, accord-
ingly mitigating the sufferer from encountering the chronic pain.
Elective techniques have risen in the previous quite a long while,
as analysts have increased a more prominent comprehension of

chronic pain and how it creates. The starting points of chronic pain are very natural: sports wounds, back wounds, fender benders - or wellbeing conditions like headaches, diabetes, joint inflammation, shingles, and malignant growth.

On occasion, notwithstanding, there is no undeniable cause of the chronic pain, no injury or injury individuals can highlight as a wellspring of their chronic pain issue - which has been baffling for the two patients and their primary care physicians

A most horrible aspect concerning this is individuals who experience chronic pain are regularly given heaps of synthetics and solutions to 'help them' feel progressively great.

This can prompt you strolling around in a fog, not so much encountering your life. All in all, what alternatives do you have - endure pain for consistently or live suddenly? Tragically, this happens to numerous competitors and dynamic people who continually experience some sort of pain. There are some elective medicines that do assist people with chronic pain.

There are options in contrast to popping pills a few times each day. Elective back pain strategies can deliver a cooling impact that truly assuages sore muscles, cramps, tired a throbbing painfulness - and that's only the tip of the iceberg. Actually, numerous world class competitors and mentors use the Alternative Pain control to help mend their hurts, pains and over-applied muscles.

The advantages to using these Alternative pain relief strategies versus different types of treatment, (for example, solutions) are many, including:

- There is no drug-instigated dimness.
- No hazardous reactions.
- You can mend your body without siphoning it brimming with synthetic substances.
- You experience quick outcomes - you don't need to stand by 30 minutes or an hour for the pain relief to produce results.
- And quite a lot more!

Individuals who experience waiting pain for quite a long time at once or even regularly are experiencing chronic pain. Because of the reactions and the potential propensity framing nature of pain prescription, huge numbers of these individuals experiencing chronic pain will refuse to take pain drug. At that point there are those individuals who just can't take medications because of hypersensitivities or different sensitivities. This is the reason in the course of recent decades chiropractic care has moved to the front of elective pain relief treatment.

With a large number of patients effectively discontent with the condition of our clinical social insurance framework, it is nothing unexpected that a huge number of individuals and patients are going to chiropractic for pain the executives and injury recovery. This is because of predictable and fruitful patient outcomes being accomplished without the use of drugs or medical procedure to advance mending. With the progression of Chiropractors' information about the sensory system, particularly in computer science, the suggestions on chiropractic care have widened enormously.

Chiropractic care is a drug free approach to address chronic pain issue by focusing on the base of the issue. The examination, finding and treatment program for clutters of the spine is performed without the use of drugs. Moreover, pain calming prescription, or some other sort of clinical need, is vital for the relief of chronic pain. Your chiropractor can elude you to a clinical specialist or doctor when required. Chiropractors work with spinal modifications and body wellbeing to accomplish similar outcomes pain medications can convey without the reactions.
Specialists of Chiropractic use a hand on approach through spinal alteration procedures and controls so as to mitigate the pain that their patients are encountering. There are many modalities your chiropractor can use to give pain relief.
Following a total examination and audit of a patient's clinical history, your chiropractor can furnish a total conclusion alongside the accessible treatment choices. A large number of the medications accessible for chronic pain relief include performing snappy push developments coordinated at a specific vertebra in the spine. Spinal altering works for chronic pain relief because it realigns the spine and decreases pressure on the nerve endings which are causing the pain somewhere else in the body.
Contingent upon the focal point of your chiropractor, the individual in question may offer a progressively all encompassing way to deal with spinal consideration. This implies they attempt to

improve a patient's general wellbeing and prosperity using great eating routine, exercise, and lifestyle directing. The conviction is that when you join sound lifestyle decisions with the normal pain relief of spinal modifying, the patient can accomplish longer enduring outcomes and keep the pain from re-happening.

CHAPTER ONE
WHAT IS PAIN? WHY DO WE EXPERIENCE IT?

Comprehend the new deduction behind chronic pain.
Let Us Ask You: What Is Pain?
It's difficult to concoct an exact definition, right? Indeed, you're not the only one. Splendid specialists, researchers, and even savants have had incredible difficulty as well. Pain has resisted scientific definition for quite a while. Sir Thomas Lewis, one of the chief British clinical researchers of the twentieth century, expressed, "I am so distant from being capable agreeably to characterize pain ... that the endeavor could fill no useful need." And Henry Ward Beecher, viewed by numerous individuals as the best American administrative speaker of his century, expressed in 1859: "... scholars and researchers have none of them prevailing with regards to characterizing pain."
In 1973, a gathering of pain specialists from around the globe met close to Seattle to talk about clinical and scientific issues in pain research and patient consideration. One of the most significant and testing errands on the motivation for this gathering of astute people was to arrive at an endless supply of pain. This gathering later developed into the esteemed International Association for the Study of Pain (IASP), which presently has in excess of 6,500 individuals from in excess of 100 nations. After much vivacious discussion and conversation, the IASP individuals concocted the following definition in 1973:

The Definition of Pain

"Pain is a horrendous tangible and enthusiastic experience related with real or potential tissue harm or depicted as far as such harm."
UNDERSTANDING THE DEFINITION OF PAIN

This meaning of pain has withstood a very long while of investigation and still remains the most acknowledged and most generally used meaning of pain today. A few significant ideas are covered up inside this apparently straightforward, one-sentence meaning of pain.

"Terrible Sensory and Emotional Experience"
In contrast to our different faculties—sight, hearing, smell, taste, and contact—the sensation of pain is constantly connected with a particularly upsetting feeling. Simply think about your past painful encounters—were any of them lovely? (We want to think not, or then you'd have another issue!)

"Genuine or Potential Tissue Damage"

When you were solicited to think from related involvements that brought about pain, you undoubtedly thought of exercises that caused a physical issue to your body, for example, a cut, a wound, a muscle sprain or strain, or maybe a wrecked bone. In fact, these would cause you to feel something you would call "pain."

Presently how about we recall the time you put your hand on that steaming hot mug of espresso and needed to immediately put the cup down on the table. In all probability, you didn't consume yourself (and subsequently encountered no injury), however it despite everything hurt like hell. It felt like you could have done some harm, right? This sort of pain is an example of "potential" substantial harm, implying that if you had not felt the consuming pain and put the cup on the table, you likely would have harmed your hand with a consume.

This is an example of what we call potential tissue injury. Also, it harms simply like genuine tissue harm, however no real injury happens.

How the pain signal goes to the brain.

The Difference between Acute and Chronic Pain

You may ask yourself: Why make a qualification between intense pain and chronic pain? The two of them hurt, isn't that right? It is imperative to recognize these sorts of pain because, despite the fact that they share much for all intents and purpose, their differences significantly affect how specialists diagnosis and treat you.

Despite the fact that the job of pain is extremely useful when intense, it is totally unseemly and counterproductive when chronic. Intense pain starts following any injury, which can be minor, for example, stubbing your toe, or major, for example, pain related with surgery or a cardiovascular failure. Regardless of whether minor or significant harm occurs, after you harm yourself a progression of substantial occasions happens. When the harm or risk is never again present, you quit feeling pain.

CHRONIC PAIN OCCURS AFTER THE HURT HAS HEALED

Chronic pain is very different. Lamentably, in all honesty, there is no generally acknowledged straightforward meaning of chronic pain. Chronic pain is characterized not just by its time course—that is, the life span of the pain following the intense injury—yet more significantly by the assurance that the recuperating procedure itself has been finished. Patients with chronic pain report that their pain is more terrible than their related knowledge with intense pain. They state that chronic pain is tiring, baffling, and endless. Intense pain is simpler to manage, truly and mentally, because you realize that it will in the long run leave. On account of chronic pain, be that as it may, there seems, by all accounts, to be no imaginable closure. Presently that harms.

The Tsunami of Chronic Pain

As expressed in the IASP's meaning of pain, pain is both a sensation and a feeling. Be that as it may, pain is significantly more mind boggling than that portrayal infers. When we take a gander at the individual pain sufferer (you) and how the pain has influenced your life, we can see that pain has an enormous undulating effect, similar to a rock tossed onto the outside of still water. Or on the other hand maybe a superior picture is one of numerous little waves that, when included, cause an incredible and damaging wave.

The tidal wave of waves causes change and stress in the lives of you and people around you, for example, work environment changes, complexities in protection, and legitimate and laborers' pay. These negative and stressful life occasions fabricate and manufacture, in the long run causing "the wave of chronic pain." You frequently feel squashed and overpowered by these issues. It appears as though regardless of where you look and regardless of what time of day it is, you are confronted with pain and all the extra stress it causes. You simply need to get the hell away!

For what reason Do We Experience Pain?

Set forth plainly, pain causes us to recall how we harmed ourselves and shows us not to do it once more. Pain causes a solid memory to engrave in our brains with the goal that we maintain a strategic distance from comparable perilous exercises later on. Pain likewise drives us to secure a harmed body part with the goal that we don't cause further injury. If we stroll on a wrecked foot, we feel more pain, so we quit doing it, along these lines forestalling further harm. Like it or not, you have to encounter pain to endure. Similarly as yearning and thirst are fundamental drives that we have to endure, we need the vibe of pain to endure. What's more, similarly as appetite and thirst are instinctual encounters that create in our brains does as well, pain. Keep in mind: Pain alerts us to genuine or potential injury.

For sure, on the frightful pain and emotions you feel inside, other unwelcome "waves" from the tidal wave show up as hindrances in your journey to discover relief. It is significant that both you and your pain specialist assess how these waves influence you. In the following areas, we will plot a portion of the intricacies (waves) and how best to oversee them.

WAVE 1: TOO MUCH LOVE FROM FRIENDS AND FAMILY

By what method can your family or companions show an excess of fondness? Through unreasonable love and mindful, they may really be aggravating your general circumstance. For example, your caring spouse might be doing all your household errands because the individual in question doesn't need you to feel more pain. A friend or family member may communicate their anxiety by not wanting you to move (because it compounds your pain). Be that as it may, by doing every one of your errands and exercises, your adored one might be coincidentally exacerbating your condition. Attempting to shield you from moving your body may cause a portion of the issues we discussed before to emerge (e.g., muscle debilitating and fit, and so forth.).

Additionally, trying to assist you with constraining your movement, companions may shun remembering you for open doors for social association, which can separate you and cause or decline depression. This lost love can turn into a major wave in the developing torrent of chronic pain.

WAVE 2: THE NEGATIVE EFFECTS ON YOUR FAMILY
Just as it wasn't awful enough as of now, the tidal wave can turn
out to be considerably progressively incredible. Frequently, your
job in the family is significantly changed. You will most likely be
unable to work and bolster your family. You will most likely be
unable to think about your more youthful, more established, or
wiped out relatives. Frequently, therefore, the pain felt by one relative is in effect "felt" by the whole family.

WAVE 3: LOSS OF SELF-ESTEEM
Alongside your powerlessness to play out your ordinary undertak-
ings comes lost confidence. You lose the pride that accompanies
the capacity to help and bolster individuals, including yourself. It
might feel just as you lose your feeling of spot right now. This
misfortune is a monster wave, adding influence to the tidal wave.

WAVE 4: THE INSURANCE, LEGAL, AND WORKERS' COM-
PENSATION SYSTEMS
Do you have a claim or laborers' pay guarantee identified with
your pain? If in this way, you are adding another colossal wave to
the torrent. Despite the fact that the huge lion's shares of chronic
pain patients who are engaged with a claim or laborers' pay case
have justifiable grievances and are not searching for an enormous
settlement, it is likely they are not being dealt with pleasantly by
the outsider in question.
Another pitiful certainty (we cautioned you there were bunches of
these) is that the legitimate and laborers' remuneration frameworks despite everything set up hindrances for the individual in
chronic pain. As a general rule, they treat you as if you are blame-
worthy until demonstrated honest. Working your way through the
protection, lawful, and laborers' pay frameworks is staggeringly
baffling and tedious. What's more, doing so just includes further
unneeded stress (of the mental sort) to your terrible circumstance.
In all honesty, if you are in such a circumstance, it is similarly as
imperative to locate an accomplished, kind, and moral legal advisor all things considered to locate a decent specialist. A decent legal counselor can significantly improve the personal satisfaction

of an individual in pain; it merits taking as much time as necessary to locate the right individual to serve you.

It is likewise critical to be careful with specialists who naturally see individuals in pain as "awful" if they have progressing claims and laborers' pay issues. Then again, you ought to be similarly careful about specialists who have been prescribed by legal counselors or associates who just observe patients with legitimate or laborers' pay issues—they might not have your wellbeing (i.e., showing signs of improvement!) on a basic level. If either of these situations is the situation, get yourself another specialist.

All Pain Is Real

You, your family, and your primary care physicians must understand that many individuals experience pain, particularly chronic pain, without having any undeniable real harm or on going potential tissue harm. Actually, all the time, chronic pain patients have totally ordinary physical examinations and research facility tests. By what means would that be able to be?

With numerous kinds of chronic pain, the standard tests don't uncover anything incorrectly or irregular in the body to clarify why the individual is encountering pain. Be that as it may, if you have chronic pain and all your lab tests are "typical," something unusual is as yet happening in your body, likely in your sensory system or muscles. An absence of examination findings doesn't suggest that the issue is "in your mind" (mental). Rather, it infers that your fundamental issue causing your pain can't be recognized by current evaluation methods specialists have accessible to them today. The tests today are basically not adequate to recognize most sensory system action—typical or strange. Keep in mind, before the approach of MRI machines, numerous patients were misdiagnosed because specialists couldn't really observe where the issue was and all the more seasoned radiology sorts of tests were ordinary. All things considered, either the clinical testing hardware today isn't sufficiently delicate to distinguish the irregularity in your body, or we, the clinical network, are still too uninformed to even consider knowing what to quantify and search for.

Break the Vicious Cycle of Chronic Pain

The Vicious Cycle of Chronic Pain (VCCP) most likely happens in definitely in excess of 90 percent of individuals with chronic pain, as a characteristic reaction to the condition. The issue is that the VCCP is terrible, exceptionally awful—it keeps you in pain, yet in addition ordinarily causes your state to exacerbate. What is the VCCP? We should talk about its essential segments.

When somebody with chronic pain moves the painful body part, the person in question ordinarily encounters an expansion in pain. This is because the patient has not been using the body part typically, coming about in:

THE BRAIN UNDER STRESS MAKES PAIN WORSE

Presently do you see why we consider it the Vicious Cycle of Chronic Pain? Within the sight of chronic pain, the uneasiness you feel with every development of your body part isn't because of extra harm, yet rather is the consequence of the advancement of tight muscles, ligaments, and tendons, and the anxiety you feel from dread. If you are not consoled by your social insurance suppliers that this pain isn't causing you more injury, it is just normal for you to accept that more harm is being finished with each sharp pain you experience during development. Your brain will then naturally turn on the stress response, which will advise you to quit moving.

Conclusion: FIND THE TREATMENT YOU DESERVE!

If your primary care physician, insurance agency, or legal counselor reveals to you the pain is all in your mind, in view of on the way that your lab tests and examinations are ordinary, if you don't mind (let us be severely legit—you should) locate an informed and prepared pain doctor to appropriately survey and treat you. For some chronic pain patients, one of the most significant things a specialist can do is to approve their pain by saying, "Indeed, the pain is genuine. Indeed, you are experiencing the pain. Truly, I will attempt to treat your pain, regardless of whether I can't identify the cause. It isn't in your mind—I trust you."

Pain Alert!

Get Educated and Get Moving! Lamentably, the horrible error of dreading development is frequently strengthened by stupid social insurance suppliers who state "If it harms, doesn't do it." With this methodology, all the more guarding and security and absence of suitable development happen, coming about in significantly increasingly musculoskeletal changes, more pain, and the inconclusive propagation of the VCCP. Thus, it is critical that you instruct yourself (as you are doing by understanding this!) and be consoled that the pain you feel with movement and active recuperation won't be destructive and is a vital piece of treatment.

CHAPTER TWO
MINDFULNESS-BASED CHRONIC
PAIN MANAGEMENT COURSES

Courses for our pain sufferers offer a significant intercession for their pain management: the opportunity to get out and meet other people who are confronting similar difficulties, and by so doing, to feel less alone and close in and different. An opportunity to impact every others' lives, focus on week by week excursions, and by analyzing our harmed lives, make sense of what should be possible, together. You will find out about a portion of their accounts right now, from a portion of their experiences, learn you are not the only one in your misery, and that your "class" is the readership of this book.

We modified the course to get as adequate as conceivable to the ordinary patient we were alluded. We were circumspect of our patients' colossal restrictions in focusing on anything, particularly week by week, and particularly as different as this was from the typical techniques, medical procedures, and drugs. In any case, we made it understood, the course was not a "rather than," it was "notwithstanding" the typical roads for some. We likewise clarified that we were not hinting that their pain was "all in their minds," or that they were here and there inadequate mentally contrasted with the individuals who mended in the ordinary time range or the individuals who didn't have chronic diseases.

No, we needed them to see that their contemplations and feelings modified their pain understanding: to be either terrible or reasonable. In turning out to be careful they could get mindful of the unfathomable connections among psyche and body. In doing as such, life may open up for them to encounter less incapacity and languishing. For a large number of the in excess of 2,000 patients who have taken our courses, it has.

As of now, we enlist chronic pain sufferers all through Ontario for our twelve-week Mindfulness-Based Chronic Pain Management (MBCPM) course. What's more, since Ontario is such a huge

Canadian region, we likewise offer classes through telemedicine to clinics in the remote zones.

In our telemedicine courses, patients living in rustic destinations go to their neighborhood emergency clinic and join our on location patients at our Toronto medical clinic area through the TV screen, so the mindfulness class is taken by patients at the same time at a few different locales and we would all be able to see one another and have conversations and reflection as though we were in a similar room.

Understanding pain mindfully

We accept that running these courses gives us a huge favorable position in understanding you as a chronic pain sufferer, as we currently spend such huge numbers of hours in conversations and contemplation in the organization of chronic pain patients. Consistently they permit us to see inside their brains and as we search around inside them with our hypothetical electric lamps, we are anxious to realize whatever they can instruct us, to comprehend the idea of pain, and to find approaches to oversee it. Enthusiastic likewise, to use this information to tell you the best way to get careful to all the more likely deal with your massively testing issue of chronic pain and inability, notwithstanding what clinical medication can offer you.

It might appear to be amazing how turning out to be progressively careful changes the manner in which a brain responds to pressure, frequently changing the pain understanding, in any event, when the pain is originating from a harmed place in the body.

One of the principal patients we had in class was a man in his mid thirties with a background marked by four back medical procedures. He had been out of the workforce for a long time and was on a moderate to high portion of opiates and other pain medications. He had driven longer than an hour to find a good pace was so doubtful during that five star that we didn't anticipate that him should return. Be that as it may, he did the day by day contemplation as mentioned, and when we showed up the next week, he had the seats previously set up for class.

Throughout the following couple of years he had a genuinely rough ride as he experienced a portion of the spirit looking through he expected to do, yet in the end he fell off his pain medications and is currently back in the workforce and getting a charge out of family life. He despite everything has pain however the pain isn't running his life any longer.

Where Is the Pain Really Coming From?

The feelings likely influence how much aggravation and nerve disturbances happen at the site of physical harm, so enthusiastic soundness adds to progressively sensible pain recognition. When we read the exploration, which shows that unusual discoveries can be found in the MRI and CT (processed tomography) outputs of the backs of individuals with no pain by any means, and that plate herniations are similarly as basic in those without back pain as in those with back pain, we start to see that we were pursuing an inappropriate analysis.
The nervous system specialist who headed the main college pain facility in which I worked in the late 1990s demanded that piece of the underlying workup ought to consistently be to discover the analysis; however back then, he truly meant discover the nerve(s) that is (are) being squeezed. It appears that, despite the fact that finding that nerve(s) is significant, the genuine determination truly includes asking: "And for what reason is there still aggravation or potentially disturbance of the nerves at that site consistently, over years not months and at times causing such extreme pain? Is the psyche, while under chronic pressure, and probably restless, empowering the steady pain messages to proceed and furthermore answerable for the poor recuperating, and if all in all, where does that reaction originate from?"

We want to show you right now this inquiry bodes well, and that it doesn't imply that you, as an individual living with chronic pain, are exclusively answerable for your powerlessness to mend, or for having a chronic pain condition.

The Mind-Body Connection

Your psyche and body are continually experiencing concoction responses occurring in a large number of cells, totally answerable for each idea you have and activity you do. Each person is one major research facility. In the kitchen, you can't get ready nour- ishment without the fixings and the cooking pots to make the concoction responses—through warmth, for instance—to make the dinner. So also, you can't move a muscle in your body without a course of synthetic responses occurring inside you that bring about that development; beginning with an inconceivably quick message from your mind, which, in itself, is because of the con- coction responses your considerations start. Your very contem- plations and feelings are compound responses.

So changing your contemplations changes those compound re- sponses, in any event, triggering changes in your safe framework, the framework you use to battle contaminations, malignant growths, and fix your harmed tissues. Maybe this data will begin to open up for you the understanding that attempting to turn out to be progressively careful, and preparing your brain to contem- plate, can really impact the remainder of your body. One impacts the other: it is classified "the brain body connection." Doing this work may even impact your reactions to your prescription.

CHAPTER THREE
PERCEIVE AND RELIEVE YOUR
CHRONIC PAIN

Beating Your Back Pain

Myofascial brokenness is the most widely recognized—and most misdiagnosed—offender.

THE PRESCRIPTION FOR BACK PAIN

Albeit a great many people dread they have a herniated (swelling) circle that will require medical procedure, most of back pain sufferers don't have a herniated plate, and regardless of whether they do they needn't bother with medical procedure.

"Undetectable" Back Pain:

A Patient's Story

I have had back pain for a long time at this point. At first, I had back medical procedure one month after I harmed my back lifting an overwhelming box grinding away. The specialist said I had a "protruding plate" that was the cause of my pain and played out a discectomy on me just about eighteen months prior, evacuating some portion of my herniated circle in my back that was seen on an attractive reverberation imaging (MRI) filter. He said the medical procedure was a triumph. Indeed, perhaps for him, however not for me! I have kept on having extreme back pain. Actually, it's more awful now than before the medical procedure. Many back specialist experts have inspected me and taken a gander at all the tests I've had both when the medical procedure—figured tomography (CT) checks, MRIs, electromyographies (EMGs), bone sweeps, and God comprehends what else. The tests have been typical, or the specialists state they see "what you hope to see after back medical procedure," so now I don't have the foggiest idea what to think. The specialist's state they can't perceive any reason why I have pain; is it all in my mind?

Along these lines, the primary medicine we keep in touch with you is to evade at first observing a back specialist who may prescribe that you go "under the knife." Also, stay away from first observing a pain management specialist who just has practical experience in nerve squares, because the individual in question will most likely suggest rehashed epidural nerve obstructs that have truly sketchy viability.

The most widely recognized guilty party in back pain is typically profound, chronic muscle fits (myofascial brokenness), which medical procedure can't help. The best solution, at that point, is multimodal treatment, for example, dynamic active recuperation (PT) joined with medications for pain that can keep you on target with the physical program. "Nontraditional" medications, for example, needle therapy and yoga likewise can help.

Medications for pain

Dynamic PT
Restorative back rub
Needle therapy
Yoga
Side effects of Back Pain

You have back pain, which, for some, individuals, stays primarily in the area of the lower back. Be that as it may, your pain may spread to your backside, hips, and legs. A great many people depict their pain as "throbbing" and "profound." Some portray it as "copying" or "sharp." If you have pain, you may feel it "shooting" and "emanating" into your legs.

Back Alert!

The Rare Neurological Warning Signs The greater part of the individuals perusing this book won't experience the accompanying admonition signs going with their back pain, yet if you do have them you need critical clinical support—no doubt medical procedure, or possibly close checking. These manifestations recommend a significant pressing of a nerve from a plate, which if not earnestly treated may cause changeless harm. Keep in mind; these are exceptionally uncommon in patients with back pain:

•   Weakness in a leg as well as foot
•   Incontinence or inconvenience peeing
•   Incontinence of stool

The vast majority with back pain have tight and delicate muscles in their lower back. When muscles are in chronic fit, they frequently cause pain where the muscles are found, yet in addition in different regions of the body, past the area of the muscles. This is called alluded pain. With low-back myofascial pain, the alluded pain can be felt in your butt, in your hips, down your leg, and into your foot, yet most people don't have eluded pain in these body districts.

Trigger points
Alluded pain territory

TRIGGER POINTS MAY CAUSE SHOOTING PAIN

Tight, delicate muscles in fit may likewise have tight bunches called myofascial trigger points, which can likewise cause alluded pain. Trigger points in your lower back can cause you to feel pain in your hip and butt cheek, or cause a shooting pain down into your leg. Most specialists are encouraged that a pain in one leg and foot is caused by sciatica, a nerve that structures close to the lower spine that is being squeezed by a swollen plate, so most will naturally expect this is the conclusion. In this manner, you can see how specialists who aren't prepared in myofascial back pain and don't analyze you for this condition will misdiagnose you with a protruding circle and pressed nerve. Tragically, this happens maybe as frequently as ninety out of multiple times, regardless of whether the patient is assessed by a decent nervous system specialist or back specialist. In all honesty, they simply don't have a clue!

Trigger points in the muscles of the hip (gluteus minimus) can cause emanating pain in the butt cheek and down the leg
Trigger Points Develop When the Sarcomeres Get Stuck
To comprehend what trigger points are and why they can grow, first you need to comprehend what makes a muscle contract. The piece of the muscle fiber that agreements are the sarcomere, which is infinitesimal in size. Each muscle contains a huge number of sarcomeres. When the sarcomeres inside a muscle consolidate as one, like when you interlock your fingers, the muscle will contract. A trigger point creates in a muscle when the sarcomeres

become harmed or are overstimulated from overuse; this causes a substance irregularity that precludes the sarcomeres from opening from their interlocked state. (This is as yet a scientific theory, and isn't yet definitively demonstrated.)

Who Gets Chronic Back Pain?
As you would envision, a ton of research has gone into attempting to address this inquiry. What the exploration found may amaze you (as it has numerous specialists, patients, and bosses): There are no organic hazard factors (e.g., being fat, having awful stance, and so forth.) for creating chronic back pain after a physical issue busy working. Except if you have had a significant herniated plate or a bit of your circle in your spinal channel has severed and is drifting in your spinal liquid (which is exceptionally uncommon), back wounds that apparently cause mellow to direct plate swell don't really cause chronic low back pain.
Considerably all the more astonishing, no specific kind of employments, for example, lifting substantial articles, make an individual bound to create back pain. In spite of the fact that you may have annoying back pain that goes back and forth If you sit excessively long in your office seat (which won't occur if you take breaks to do some extending exercises!), you won't create chronic crippling back pain except if you have a specific significant hazard factor!
The factor that has been identified to put individuals in danger of creating chronic back pain is an absence of fulfillment and power over one's occupation. The business related injury doesn't need to be extreme; the pain can be caused by a minor curving of the back or by lifting a couple of books or reams of paper.
As it were, if you are distraught in your activity and you have a feeling that your supervisor is a micromanaging rascal, or you don't feel esteemed for the work you do, you might be in danger of creating chronic back pain. Tragically, some exploration shows that numerous if not a great many people are unsettled or fulfilled in their employments, which may clarify why the condition is so normal! What's more, particularly with the present economy the manner in which it has been, an ever increasing number of individuals will be taking occupations they don't discover fulfilling and will be in danger of creating chronic low back pain.
Back Pain is a Common Problem

Back pain is nearly as broad as the normal virus. Studies have indicated that every one of us has around a 75 percent possibility of encountering back pain at some point during our life. This part will help you if you have back pain now, yet in addition set up us all for the future and help any friends and family who are presently experiencing this condition. Right now, will speak for the most part about chronic back pain that has gone on for a while and is situated in the lumbar district, the least piece of your back. As we stated, the most widely recognized cause of this pain is chronic muscle fit, additionally called myofascial brokenness. We have all had intense muscle fits, in which a muscle immediately agreements or issues, causing sharp, consuming, cutting, and additionally throbbing pain at the site of the fit. Myofascial brokenness happens when a muscle or gathering of muscles (just as tendons and ligaments) gets arranged to out of nowhere going into a fit or spasm chronically. There might be times when the muscle is loose, however whenever it might get broken and go into a fit or squeezing mode.

Trigger points in the back and neck
Every delicate tissue (muscles, tendons, and ligaments) can go into a chronic condition of touchiness to fit and squeezing because of injury or injury, medical procedure, or monotonous use, disuse, or misuse. Like bunches of our body parts, we underestimate our muscles, tendons, and ligaments for conceded; if we use them to an extreme or excessively little, they can go into an anomalous state and apparently fight their misuse! Fortunately, however, when we figure out how to use them appropriately, the muscles can without much of a stretch return into their cheerful, nonpainful state.

Medications to Treat Back Pain

Albeit no drug genuinely acts to assuage the muscle fit at the wellspring of most people's back pain, a wide range of kinds of medications can ease the pain you feel. Medications can improve your personal satisfaction and streamline the impacts of PT. There truly is anything but a "best" medicine; rather, your primary care physician ought to recommend the drugs on an experimentation premise, first using the ones with minimal number of conceivable symptoms.

NSAIDS AND COX-2 INHIBITORS REDUCE INFLAMMATION
Now and again, patients do discover relief from the anti-inflammatory and general pain-mitigating impacts of nonsteroidal anti-inflammatory drugs (NSAIDs, for example, Voltaren, Motrin, and Aleve) and COX-2 inhibitor medications (Celebrex) when taken orally as pills, tablets, and containers. Be that as it may, these normally offer just slight to direct relief, best case scenario. Likewise, these medications can cause conceivably genuine reactions if devoured too much of the time or at too high a portion, regardless of whether purchased as over-the-counter (OTC) arrangements. If taken erroneously, they can cause genuine liver, kidney, and heart issues. Be that as it may, if taken as suggested, these medications can be useful for some individuals. For more data on how they work, see "Medications to Treat OA Pain,".

If one of these medications doesn't give you enough relief or gives you deplorable symptoms—the most well-known being vexed stomach—it's advantageous to attempt a couple of others to discover one that gives you important pain relief without terrible symptoms, as everybody will respond differently to each.

TOPICAL NSAIDS HAVE FEWER SIDE EFFECTS
In the United States, topical NSAID arrangements, for example, Pennsaid, Voltaren Gel, and Flector Patch have as of late been FDA-endorsed for treating certain chronic pain conditions, for example, joint inflammation and intense games injury pain. In spite of the fact that they have
not been tried to treat chronic musculoskeletal pain, all things considered, these moisturizers, creams, and fixes may deliver comparative pain relief as a similar drug taken orally, however with less possibility of building up the reactions related with ingesting pills or containers. These kinds of drugs, accessible in Europe and Asia for quite a few years, have a similar medication found in oral NSAIDs, however produce lower measures of the drug in the blood because they act locally, and in this manner hypothetically lessen the dangers for genuine and irksome reactions. For topical NSAIDs, the prescribed application for Pennsaid and Voltaren Gel is four times each day straightforwardly to the site of

pain. The prescribed portion for the Flector Patch, a topical NSAID, is one fix like clockwork.

Pill Alert!

Secure Your Medications to Reduce Drug Abuse! A great deal of media consideration has been focused on narcotic (opiate) medications as of late because of the significant cultural issue of passings related with the misuse of these drugs. The significant wellspring of misuse is from youngsters taking them from their family's medication bureau. You can keep this from occurring by keeping these medications in a sheltered and ensured zone of your house. Likewise, if you have additional pills from a remedy that you are finished with, discard them! For the earth and water supply, don't flush them down the latrine, but instead blend them in with espresso beans or feline litter and put them in the trash. Try not to save them for the future; numerous individuals "squirrel them away," figuring they may require them sometime in the not so distant future. Try not to store them. Dispose of them and spare a life!

THE LIDOCAINE PATCH 5% (LIDODERM) REDUCES PAIN

Despite the fact that the lidocaine fix isn't FDA-endorsed to treat back pain, a few distributed investigations have demonstrated that a few patients with back pain report excellent relief and no genuine reactions from applying up to four lidocaine fixes legitimately to their lower back area. (Lidoderm is just FDA-affirmed to treat chronic nerve pain after shingles, a condition called postherpetic neuralgia.)

The FDA-endorsed dosing for lidocaine fix 5% is up to three fixes at a time applied to the painful zone for twelve hours on and afterward twelve hours off. Be that as it may, numerous examinations have been distributed demonstrating that it is sheltered to use up to four fixes at once, keeping them on for twenty-four hours and afterward putting on new fixes.

TRAMADOL COMBINES TWO MECHANISMS

Tramadol is a fascinating drug with a few different pain-easing systems, including going about as a feeble narcotic (at times called opiate) joined with the capacity to take a shot at the synthetic substances norepinephrine and serotonin that have been appeared to assist produce with paining relief in the spinal line and cerebrum. A few decent examinations show that a few patients with back pain experience significant pain relief with tramadol and without insufferable symptoms. Tramadol is currently accessible both as a long-acting once-per-day pill (Ryzolt and Ultram ER) just as quick discharge pills taken four times each day (Ultram and generics). One accessible arrangement of tramadol is joined with acetaminophen (Ultracet).

DULOXETINE (CYMBALTA) WORKS IN THE SPINE AND BRAIN
As of late, scientific preliminaries have indicated that duloxetine can create generally excellent pain relief in patients with back pain. Duloxetine takes a shot at two synapse synthetics associated with the view of pain in the spinal rope and mind, norepinephrine and serotonin. It is accessible as a pill and is frequently taken once day by day.

Narcotics *ARE CAUTIOUSLY RECOMMENDED FOR CERTAIN PATIENTS*

Narcotic medicine (opiates) has as of late been demonstrated to be of advantage for certain individuals experiencing moderate to extreme back pain. Like all medications used in treating back pain, narcotics are not a fix, yet when endorsed fittingly they can improve the odds of a functioning PT program being fruitful.
As we would see it, narcotics ought not routinely be recommended as first-line medicine for some patients with back pain because of their potential for reactions, the uncommon danger of habit, and the potential for misuse and preoccupation (somebody taking your pills for a high or to sell for cash) of these kinds of medications. In any case, for certain patients, narcotic prescription can significantly expand personal satisfaction and can mean the difference among progress and disappointment with the required PT program. It is indispensable that you use all medications as recommended to boost both their pain soothing advantage just as your security.

What's going on: FDA Approvals for Back Pain?
Tapentadol (showcased as Nucynta), like tramadol, follows up on two synthetic substances in the spinal rope and mind: the sedative framework and the neurochemical norepinephrine, the two synapses that we normally have in our body that have been

demonstrated to be associated with our regular pain-soothing pathways. Tapentadol has been appeared in studies to mitigate low back pain and different kinds of chronic pain (and intense pain). It is presently accessible just as a short-acting, quick discharge pill, however an all-inclusive discharge pill is being worked on.

Tanezumab is being created by the pharmaceutical organization Pfizer to treat different kinds of chronic pain. This is really a novel kind of drug, as it attempts to hinder the protein nerve development factor that has a major impact in the improvement of pain after injury and aggravation. As this book went to press, tanezumab had a significant setback as the FDA raised worries about the potential security of this drug, particularly in patients with osteoarthritis. If it in the long run gets FDA endorsement, patients will probably be required to infuse tanezumab each eight to twelve weeks for treatment to be fruitful.

Nonmedication Therapies for Back Pain Relief

We emphatically accept these are a higher priority than drug treatment (or infusions, gadgets, or medical procedure) for most by far of individuals with back pain. The accompanying kinds of treatments mean to diminish the chronic muscle fits and tight/delicate tendons and ligaments related with back pain, and are essential in mitigating the indications identified with this condition.

If you experience the ill effects of this very normal clinical issue, you should locate an accomplished pain expert who can perform one of these treatments (or a blend) to focus on the core of your concern and really resolve your fits and back pain. What's more, recollect, because a specialist has "Pain Management" alongside their name doesn't mean the individual realizes how to suitably assess and treat back pain. The well-known axiom "If the sum total of what you have is a sledge, everything seems as though a nail" is valid with specialists as well; a back specialist is destined to prescribe back medical procedure and an interventional pain management expert is destined to suggest nerve squares whether you genuinely need them or not.

Back Alert!

Work through the Initial Pain With fruitful dynamic PT, it is normal that pain may deteriorate during the underlying stages before it shows signs of improvement. This is because the muscles at the center of your concern have become accustomed to being in a spastic state, so at first, moving them can cause them to go into further fit, and subsequently can cause more pain. In any case, you ought to understand that indeed, this underlying exacerbating of your pain is a decent sign because it implies the muscles liable for your back pain are the ones getting the required treatment.

We've seen such a large number of patients use pain as their guide for day by day movement levels. That is, on the "acceptable days" they try too hard, and on the "awful days" they become habitually lazy people. Suppose Monday and Tuesday were terrible pain days, so you remained in bed or on the lounge chair for the greater part of the day. Wednesday was a pleasant, radiant day and your pain was better, so you attempted to achieve two days of exercises to compensate for some recent setbacks. And afterward learn to expect the unexpected. On Thursday, you were back in bed and on the sofa. Does this sound recognizable? This isn't reasonable!

You ought to do a similar measure of action and exercise each day, paying little mind to your pain level. For example, if you have not been dynamic at all for a while, you should begin little—state, two to five minutes of delicate exercise every day. At that point each seven to fourteen days, bit by bit increment the measure of exercise by 5 percent to 10 percent, again paying little heed to your pain level. The key message is to take it "gradual," and not to base your degree of day by day movement and exercise on the measure of pain you are feeling that day.

DYNAMIC PHYSICAL THERAPY (PT) IS PARAMOUNT

All pain management specialists concur that a functioning PT program is the most significant treatment for patients with back pain that isn't because of plate sickness. This for the most part alludes to a program that includes the patient steadily expanding the use of applicable muscles through extending, reinforcing, and continuance exercises. Your program will empower you to steadily build how regularly and for what timeframe you can use the muscles that are causing your back pain.

It is significant that patients with back pain work with a physical specialist who has been prepared to treat this condition. Again and again, undeveloped physical advisors will treat all back pain patients a similar way, which is with "inactive" modalities, for example, rub, heat packs, and ultrasound, bringing about wrong treatment and imperfect outcomes. By identifying the specific muscles at the center of your back pain, the physical advisor can structure a custom fitted exercise and restorative program that trains in on your fundamental issue.

ACUPUNCTURE THERAPY IS SAFE AND MAY BE BENEFICIAL
Many back pain patients report significant pain relief with a progression of needle therapy medicines performed by a prepared acupuncturist. In spite of the fact that scientific examinations have indicated blended outcomes (both positive and negative) with this type of treatment, it is our assessment that needle therapy can be a safe and conceivably exceptionally accommodating treatment for enough back pain patients that it might be considered.
TRIGGER-POINT INJECTIONS RELEASE THE KNOTS
Trigger-point infusions (TPIs) are exactly what the name suggests: infusions made legitimately into the tight, spastic district of the muscle. TPIs should be possible by means of a few different strategies, including simply embeddings a needle therapy needle (additionally called dry-needling), infusing lidocaine or another neighborhood sedative drug, infusing a steroid, or infusing a nearby sedative with a steroid. In our view, there is no genuine favorable position to infusing any drug into the trigger point (aside from maybe botulinum poison, otherwise called BOTOX, MY-BLOC or DYSPORT); be that as it may, a few patients guarantee they experience less pain and uneasiness with the intense pain related with TPI if lidocaine or another neighborhood sedative is infused into the trigger point. TPIs can work for a considerable length of time, weeks, or even a very long time to ease pain and increment development.
It isn't clear how frequently TPIs ought to be given. Most pain specialists suggest an underlying preliminary of week after week TPIs for four to about a month and a half, and afterward

rethinking to check whether the patient is encountering a positive result. Once more, it is fundamentally significant that during this TPI preliminary, the patient is likewise joined up with a functioning PT program.

WARMTH TREATMENT OFFERS SHORT-TERM RELIEF

In the course of recent years, we have seen a showcasing push to treat a wide range of pain, including back pain, with an applied warmth wrap (e.g., the OTC warmth wrap ThermaCare). There is some proof that heat-wrap treatment can give a little level of momentary pain relief in patients with back pain.

A comparable treatment for back pain is the utilization of a focused warmth source legitimately at the myofascial trigger points; this is alluded to as central warmth trigger-point (FHTP) treatment. This treatment demonstrations like a TPI, however isn't obtrusive and the patient can do it at home.

One such FHTP gadget, Zeno, is an OTC treatment for skin inflammation that we've used to give TPIs some achievement.

CRANIOSACRAL THERAPY WORKS FOR SOME

A few patients with myofascial pain report significant pain relief and improved capacity with craniosacral treatment. These kinds of medications ought to be performed via prepared advisors with involvement with treating patients with chronic pain.

Back Alert!

Drawbacks to TPIs The initial not many TPIs you get can be very painful. The muscle may really go into more profound fits before it in the long run relearns how to unwind. The key with myofascial TPIs is that the patient all the while takes part in a functioning PT program. Notwithstanding potential drawbacks, patients with back pain ought to genuinely consider TPIs from an accomplished doctor as a sheltered treatment to help ease the indications of their condition.

RESTORATIVE MASSAGE AND ACUPRESSURE MAY ALSO WORK

Some proof recommends that restorative back rub and pressure point massage treatment may demonstrate useful in certain patients with back pain. Once more, these treatments ought to be matched with a functioning PT/exercise program. Additionally, it is significant not to simply get an extraordinary body knead at your neighborhood spa, yet rather to locate a restorative back rub specialist who realizes how to treat back pain.

DELICATE YOGA INCREASES STRENGTH AND FLEXIBILITY

There are various kinds of yoga, some delicate and others all the more requesting. The back pain sufferer should locate a delicate kind of yoga, for example, hatha yoga. Hatha yoga is a moderate paced extending class with some straightforward breathing exercises and reflections typically done in a situated position. An ongoing investigation of yoga and chronic back pain found that following twelve weeks of yoga, 73 percent of the yoga bunch said they had by and large improvement in back pain, as contrasted and 27 percent of the benchmark group that kept on observing their primary care physician and take their prescribed medications.

CHIROPRACTORS ARE CAUTIOUSLY RECOMMENDED

Despite the fact that chiropractic medications are one of the more typical medicines individuals look for when they have back pain, we need to caution you that we just carefully suggest such treatment. Studies have indicated that chiropractic controls can help improve the side effects of back pain; however there is a potential danger of genuine injury if you don't have an "ordinary" back (see sidebar "Before You See a Chiropractor"). Likewise with any human services professional treating your condition, it is significant that the chiropractor be very much experienced in treating chronic back pain.

Chiropractic medication depends on the conviction that the spine may have confined development that prompts pain and poor capacity. When a chiropractor "controls" your back (likewise called spinal change), the individual in question will apply an abrupt power to your back bones, pushing or pulling the vertebrae to different unnatural positions. This utilization of power is the thing that causes the popping and breaking sounds you hear exuding

from their workplaces! On occasion, a chiropractor may likewise use rub and delicate extending strategies too.
Back Alert!

Before You See a Chiropractor It is significant that your analysis of myofascial back pain be made by a prepared back pain doctor before you see a chiropractor. If your back pain is really originating from genuine plate illness, a portion of the chiropractic controls performed could bring about genuine neurological harm.

STRESS MANAGEMENT TECHNIQUES REDUCE TENSION

The pressure response has been appeared to cause compounding muscle fits, particularly in muscles that are inclined to fit (myofascial brokenness). Along these lines, it bodes well that pressure management systems, for example, unwinding, symbolism, and biofeedback, would all be able to assume a significant job in the treatment of back pain.
MENTAL TREATMENTS RELIEVE THE MIND AND BACK

Many back pain patients create sorrow because of their steady, persistent, crippling pain. If this transpires, you should look for mental treatment. Studies have demonstrated that patients with a wide range of chronic pain and wretchedness or nervousness will be less receptive to their pain medicines if these mental conditions are not likewise treated. Back pain patients who may have a mental condition, for example, sadness, uneasiness, or post-awful pressure issue, ought to be assessed by a specialist or therapist. Contingent upon the seriousness of your condition, the person may suggest a straightforward course of antidepressant drug as well as different kinds of mental treatments, for example, subjective social treatment.
Feeling Depressed Is Par for the Course
Try not to be embarrassed if you have one of these mental conditions because of your back pain. Pretty much every patient we have treated with chronic back pain has sooner or later during their sickness created sadness or another mental condition because of how their life has been adversely influenced by their back pain.

Treatments That Do Not Work For Back Pain

"MUSCLE RELAXANTS" ARE REALLY SEDATIVES

In spite of the fact that numerous drugs have been advertised as "muscle relaxants," they don't really loosen up the muscles! Truth be told, no drug has been appeared to significantly diminish the fit of chronic myofascial pain conditions. Or maybe, muscle relaxer drugs likely work also to Valium and "unwind" your muscles just by quieting you. When you're snoozing, you normally loosen up your muscles—however you can't live in a quieted express as long as you can remember, in spite of what that infectious Ramones tune says!

Back Alert!

No Case for Nerve Blocks

We accept there is no job for a progression of nerve hinders in the treatment of chronic back pain except if obviously the cause of your chronic back pain has been demonstrated to be receptive to nerve squares. Most regularly, "being responsive" signifies giving a perceptible level of pain relief for a time of weeks to months. Continue circumspectly if you are guaranteed 100 percent pain relief for eternity! We've seen an excessive number of patients go to nerve square shops (specialists and centers that treat all types of pain with just nerve squares) and get many infusions with no long haul great outcomes, just to stop these medicines with no adjustment in their pain yet with an a lot lighter wallet. Be careful with "pain specialists" who just skill to treat pain with a sharp needle focused on your back!

DETACHED PT FEELS GOOD ONLY BRIEFLY

Many—if not most—physical specialists are prepared in just inactive, "feel better" treatments, for example, steaming showers, delicate back rub, and ultrasound. Ultrasound is a system wherein sound waves are applied to the muscles of your back in order to get them to unwind. In spite of the fact that these kinds of PT procedures feel incredible when you get them, they won't treat, resolve, or fix your back issue.

Medical procedure is not warranted for back pain from spasms

There is positively no job for medical procedure in the treatment of chronic back pain because of muscle fit. We have seen awfully numerous patients with back pain who need a convenient solution and would like to discover a specialist who is happy to do back medical procedure on them.

Not exclusively does this not help, yet frequently it exacerbates the pain and incapacity. Kindly doesn't be one of these people!

SPINAL CORD STIMULATION IS A COSTLY LAST RESORT

Despite the fact that proof proposes that spinal rope incitement might be good for certain patients with different sorts of back pain, it is our conclusion that this costly kind of treatment should regularly be held if all else fails for patients with back pain. Here, as well, be careful with pain experts who regularly just addition spinal line triggers for a wide range of pain. A portion of these specialists amass a lot of riches from these methods, so they rush to prescribe this kind of treatment.

Diagnosing Back Pain

To start with, to analyze the cause of your back pain, you'll have to have a nervous system specialist, a physical medication/restoration specialist, or an appropriately prepared essential consideration specialist assess you. These sorts of specialists will be authorities in the examination of the nerves in your spine, and hence can survey your back for any potential related neurological variations from the norm. Similarly as with most patients with back pain, your neurological examination will probably be typical (if not, see the Back Alert! about notice signs).

Second, after finishing a myofascial examination, the specialist will probably discover muscle trigger points that imitate your pain when palpated and delicately squeezed. That is it; no "extravagant schmancy" costly tests required!

The back has numerous muscles, all of which may have trigger points

Back Alert!

Baseless Surgeries Cause Problems When we were youthful pain specialists and patients returned to us after medical procedure still in pain, we thought we were seeing just a one-sided test; that perhaps there were numerous fruitful back medical procedures and we were seeing just the individuals who didn't progress nicely. Sadly, that doesn't seem, by all accounts, to be the situation. An excessive number of people are encouraged to experience back medical procedure when they needn't bother with it, and a significant number of them are getting medical procedures, for example, combinations, that produce a large group of new issues that are difficult if not difficult to treat without more medical procedure. Be careful!

FINDING MYOFASCIAL TRIGGER POINTS

Despite the fact that diagnosing myofascial trigger points isn't advanced science, sadly most specialists aren't prepared to play out a legitimate assessment for trigger points, and may not know about what a trigger point is.

Examination Findings: Back Pain

The neurological examination in patients with back pain because of muscle fit is totally ordinary. In any case, unmistakable anomalies are found on the myofascial examination of the muscles of the lower back. When the specialist surveys the muscles for trigger points, the individual will find that softly pushing on the tight and delicate muscles will be painful and can mirror the patient's pain symptoms. Regularly, tenderly pushing on these tight muscles will cause the patient's pain to spread (e.g., into the butt cheek and down into the leg).

To discover a myofascial trigger point, a specialist ought to tenderly rub their fingers along your muscles, tendons, and ligaments and feel for tight, hard bunches, and afterward delicately and slowly push these tight bunches with their thumb to see your response. We as a whole have trigger points at different occasions. To make a diagnosis of myofascial back pain, the trigger points in your back area, when squeezed, should cause you to have a specific response.

To start with, myofascial trigger points liable for your pain may cause what's known as a jerk reaction, which means the specialist can feel the muscle, ligament, or tendon really jerk. Second, you will feel pain that copies the pain you feel precipitously. Third, you may likewise feel alluded pain, so you will feel pain where the specialist is squeezing, yet additionally in a different area. For example, trigger points in muscles along the lower back area can cause you to feel pain in your hip, butt cheek, and even leg. Because specialists aren't regularly prepared in trigger points, they erroneously analyze pain that begins in the back and shoots into your butt cheek or leg as "sciatica," caused by a swelling plate that is aggravating or crushing a nerve root leaving your spine. That is the reason it's fundamentally significant that you be inspected by an accomplished and proficient specialist.

NO LAB TESTS NEEDED TO DIAGNOSE MOST BACK PAIN

Radiology tests, for example, X-beams, CT sweeps, and MRIs, don't give the cause to most by far of patients with back pain. Strangely, notwithstanding, an ongoing report from Stanford University demonstrated that regions of the United States with the most noteworthy number of MRIs likewise have the most elevated number of medical procedures for low back pain, with the senior researcher finishing up, "The net outcome is expanded dangers of superfluous medical procedure for patients and expanded expenses for every other person."

Electromyograms (EMG) and nerve conduction (NCV) tests might possibly exhibit unusual muscle fit, yet they don't show any nerve harm. EMG/NCV tests are regularly totally typical in people with back pain.

What's in store from a Neurological Examination?

For all chronic pain conditions, your primary care physician ought to play out an exhaustive neurological examination, which has three fundamental parts:

Engine: The specialist will have you push and pull your different muscles to assess their quality.

Tangible: The specialist will test your tactile recognition as different items contact your body; each article assesses different nerves and parts of your sensory system. These incorporate delicately scouring a finger or a Q-tip over your skin, jabbing you with a pin (you should state "ouch"), and putting a vibrating tuning fork on your toe and finger joints, and inquiring as to whether you feel a vibration.

Reflexes: The specialist will take out their trusty reflex sledge and check your reflexes at your knee, yet additionally at your lower legs, elbow, and wrist.

Less Common Causes of Back Pain

In spite of the fact that by a long shot the most well-known cause of chronic back pain is muscle fit and the vast majority are generally dreadful of having a herniated plate, there are different less normal issues you ought to know about:

CHAPTER FOUR
SPONDYLOLISTHESIS

What's going on here? Spondylolisthesis happens when the vertebral bone in the lower some portion of the spine slips forward and onto the vertebra below it.

Diagnosis:

• Diagnosis is effectively made through a straightforward plain X-beam of the lower back.

Symptoms:
• Pain is felt in the lower back, and potentially in the posterior and hips.
• The back feels stiff.
• Tenderness is felt in the area of the slipped vertebra.

Treatment:

• For most patients, the treatment is like that for myofascial back pain.
• Patients with serious pain or extreme slippage that doesn't react to traditionalist treatment may expect medical procedure to fuse the vertebral bones together.

SPINAL STENOSIS

What's going on here? Spinal stenosis is a narrowing of the focal trench (opening) in which the spine nerves travel.

Diagnosis:
• On examination, patients with lumbar (low back) stenosis regularly have shortcoming and some anomalous sensations in their legs, which they may not by any means notice. Patients with cervical (neck) stenosis have shortcoming and anomalous sensations in their arms, hands, or fingers.
• Laboratory tests, for example, MRI/CT outputs and plain X-beams show narrowing of the spinal trench.

• EMG may likewise help make the diagnosis.

Symptoms:
For lower back spinal stenosis:
• Commonly, patients whine of pain or squeezing in their legs with delayed standing or strolling, which rapidly improves with twisting around or plunking down.
• Pain may spread into the legs.
• Patients may encounter deadness and shivering in the legs.
For neck spinal stenosis:

• Patients experience pain and squeezing in the shoulders, arms, and legs.
• The hands are ungainly.
• Sometimes inconvenience strolling and terrible parity can likewise happen.
Treatment:
This condition is significantly more typical in the low back than in the neck district
• Again, all patients ought to at first attempt nonsurgical treatments for in any event three months, including dynamic PT and medicine.
• If preservationist treatment fizzles, epidural nerve squares might be attempted before medical procedure.
• As a final retreat, medical procedure might be expected to build the initial where the sickness procedure has limited the waterway.
ANKYLOSING SPONDYLITIS

What's going on here? This is a chronic inflammatory joint pain and auto-resistant condition that in the long run may cause strange spine and pelvis bone development and combination of the bones. This condition is significantly more typical in the low back than in the neck locale. It is accepted to be an acquired hereditary issue.
Diagnosis:
• In later stages, plain X-beams and MRI/CT sweeps can show anomalies.

• Blood tests can be useful to exhibit a strange inflammatory procedure, for example, erythrocyte sedimentation rate and C-responsive protein (CRP).

• Genetic testing for the HLA-B27 quality can likewise be used to analyze this condition.

Symptoms:

• In beginning periods, this condition may mirror myofascial back pain.

• As the malady advances, symptoms spread to conceivably incorporate stiffness of the whole spine and a failure to take full breaths (rib inclusion).

- An indication is if you create eye pain or obscured vision, as the eye may become engaged with the infection procedure.

• When A.S. includes the neck, which aren't normal, symptoms incorporate neck pain and stiffness with loss of neck development.

Treatment:

Here is the place specific medications can significantly affect the malady procedure. These drugs include:

• NSAIDs

• Disease-modifying antirheumatic drugs, for example, sulfasalazine or methotrexate. These may assist with restricting the aggravation and harm. Notwithstanding, there are potential genuine symptoms of low blood tallies and liver harm that should be checked during treatment with these drugs.

• Corticosteroids. When recommended chronically, these may likewise assist with diminishing the inflammatory procedure and limit harm in extreme cases, as back pain is one of the uncommon conditions in which the advantages of chronic steroid use may exceed the dangers.

• Tumor rots factor blockers, for example, adalimumab (Humira), etanercept (Enbrel), and infliximab (Remicade). These are moderately new kinds of drugs that obstruct a specific protein answerable for irritation. These drugs would all be able to have genuinely sensational positive outcomes, yet in addition have the potential for intense symptoms, including contaminations, for example, tuberculosis, seizures, or aggravation of the nerves of the eyes, intensifying of cardiovascular breakdown, a lupus-like disorder, and lymphoma, a sort of disease.

Getting a Grip on Neck Pain

The ideal remedy is multimodal treatment, where the most basic treatment is an active exercise based recuperation (PT) program. Prescription can diminish the pain to make the PT program increasingly profitable. Moreover, "nontraditional" treatments, for example, acupuncture can help. Likewise, huge numbers of the mental treatments talked about right now have a major effect for some patients with neck pain.

Medications for pain
Active PT
Nontraditional treatments, for example, acupuncture
Brain research
Symptoms of Neck Pain
You have neck pain, most ordinarily depicted by patients as profound, hurting, consuming, and sharp. For a great many people, the pain spreads past their neck, so it shouldn't be astonishing if your pain shoots into your shoulders and arms or is joined by a migraine. Numerous patients with neck pain likewise whine of feeling mixed up and bleary eyed. This is because the muscles in the neck really assume a job in keeping our bodies adjusted (with the goal that we don't fall) by telling our cerebrum the area of our head. Consequently, when these muscles go into fit, they can give the mind falsehood and cause a sentiment of dazedness.

Much like chronic back pain, there are numerous causes of neck pain. Also, as back pain, time after time individuals are told (or self-analyze) that their pain is because of a plate swell, a squeezed nerve in the neck, or joint pain. More often than not this is off base. Truth be told, the most well-known cause of neck pain, as back pain, is drawn out tight and spastic muscles (myofascial pain).

Pain Alert!

Trigger Point or Disk Bulge

Muscles, tendons, and ligaments all can be influenced by myofascial brokenness and grow tight, delicate central regions, or what you may call "tight bunches." These delicate locales of your muscles, tendons, or ligaments are called trigger points.

Trigger points cause pain locally, yet in addition—or some of the time just—in territories that are inaccessible from the trigger point (known as alluded pain). Trigger points in certain neck muscles can cause you to have pain in your shoulder and arm and can even cause pressure type cerebral pains. If you are a headache sufferer, they may welcome on one of these migraines.

Thusly, you and your primary care physician must understand that because the pain may shoot from your neck and into your arms doesn't really mean the pain is from a plate swell or from a nerve root being pressed in the neck. Numerous specialists expect this is the situation, prompting an off-base diagnosis and wrong treatment, and once in a while even ridiculous neck medical procedure. Be cautious!

Medications for Neck Pain

NSAIDS/COX-2 INHIBITORS RELIEVE PAIN

Now and again, a few patients do discover slight to direct relief using remedy quality nonsteroidal anti-inflammatory drugs (NSAIDs) and COX-2 inhibitor medications. These medications decrease irritation and furthermore can have an immediate pain-alleviating impact. It is critical to consider the potential genuine symptoms of these drugs, regardless of whether purchased over the counter. If taken again and again or at too high a portion, they can cause significant liver, kidney, and heart issues. Be that as it may, for certain patients, these medications can give great pain relief without terrible symptoms, when taken as suggested. Peruse the name and follow the suggested dosing.
Neck Alert!

Enjoy a Reprieve from the Computer Here's a straightforward procedure to lighten and forestall neck pain, proposed by a pain analyst: Put a red dab on your PC or console as a suggestion to take a little break each ten to fifteen minutes to extend your neck and back and do some profound breathing exercises. This routine can really forestall neck and back pain, and offer your eyes a reprieve also!

THE LIDOCAINE PATCH 5% WORKS ON THE SPOT
Despite the fact that it isn't FDA-endorsed to treat neck pain, a few patients have announced getting some pain relief with Lidoderm. Lidocaine, the active medication in Lidoderm, acts legitimately on pain nerves in the skin and muscles to calm down the force of the pain signals they are delivering. Because Lidoderm is a topical drug, there are no known genuine symptoms and no drug collaborations to stress over. The FDA-endorsed dosing for lidocaine fix 5% is up to three fixes at a time applied to the painful territory twelve hours on and afterward twelve hours off. In any case, numerous examinations have been distributed demonstrating that it is sheltered to use up to four fixes at once, keeping them on for twenty-four hours and afterward putting on new fixes.

TOPICAL NSAIDS HAVE MINIMAL SERIOUS SIDE EFFECTS

Despite the fact that not read for the treatment of neck pain, topical NSAID medications are much of the time used outside the United States for treating neck pain. Because these are topical drugs, there are no known genuine reactions and no drug associations to be worried about; with the exception of once in a while all diclofenac items may cause liver anomalies. These drugs legitimately infuse anti-inflammatory operators into the aggravated muscles, tendons, and ligaments. Topical NSAIDs are not FDA-endorsed to treat neck pain, however they are affirmed to treat osteoarthritis and intense minor games injury pain. Right now FDA-affirmed and accessible topical NSAID salves and gels are applied multiple times day by day to the painful area; the proposal for the Flector Patch is one fix day by day, to be supplanted by another fix.

Neck Alert!

Be "Smart Active" When Your Pain Isn't Bad When you discover a prescription that mitigates your neck pain, it is significant that you use the without pain periods to participate in the PT treatments that will find a good pace of the issue.

TRAMADOL WORKS IN TWO WAYS

Tramadol is a fascinating drug with two different pain-easing components in the spine and cerebrum: one on the sensory system's narcotic framework and the other on the synapses norepinephrine and serotonin. A few decent examinations show that a few patients with back pain experience significant pain relief with tramadol, without horrendous reactions. Hence, it is likely neck pain patients may get relief from tramadol also.

NARCOTICS ARE CAUTIOUSLY RECOMMENDED TO CERTAIN PATIENTS

Narcotic drug can profit certain sufferers of neck pain. Like all medications for this condition, narcotics are not a fix, yet when recommended fittingly for the right patient they can enable a patient to take an interest in a required active PT program. Narcotics work by straightforwardly connecting with common narcotic frameworks in the spinal string and cerebrum and furthermore likely on the fringe nerves. They ought not be endorsed as first-line treatment because of their inclination for causing symptoms and because of the uncommon events of compulsion and preoccupation (somebody taking your pills for a high or to sell for cash). In any case, for patients who are seriously weakened from their neck pain and for whom nothing else has worked, narcotics can be a gift from heaven.

Nonmedication Therapies for Neck Pain

Following are the most significant treatments in treating neck pain caused by myofascial issues; the most widely recognized cause of neck pain. At least one of these is totally important to find a good pace and really resolve the issue causing the pain.

ACTIVE PT IS NUMBER ONE

An active PT program is by a long shot the most significant treatment for patients with neck pain. The most significant objective of this treatment is for the patient to step by step increment the use of the included neck muscles with extending, fortifying, and continuance exercises.

When starting a PT program, anticipate that the pain should deteriorate during the initial scarcely any meetings. Realize that this declining is a decent sign, as it implies the muscles answerable for your chronic pain are the ones accepting the required treatment.

ACUPUNCTURE CAN PROVIDE SIGNIFICANT RELIEF

Many neck pain patients get significant pain relief with a progression of acupuncture treatments performed by a prepared acupuncturist. In spite of the fact that reviews need substantial proof, we prescribe acupuncture as a safe and conceivably accommodating treatment for neck pain because we've seen generally excellent outcomes in certain patients. Nobody really knows how acupuncture functions, however Chinese medication claims it controls hidden energies, a hypothesis inconsequential to our Western medication's anatomical and physiological precepts and convictions.

TRIGGER POINT INJECTIONS (TPIs) FIND THE TROUBLE SPOT

TPIs are exactly what the name infers—infusions pointed straightforwardly into the tight, spastic locale of the muscle. Contingent upon specialist inclination, TPIs should be possible by using an acupuncture needle (additionally called dry-needling), or by infusing a neighborhood sedative, for example, lidocaine, a steroid, or both a nearby sedative and a steroid. As far as we can tell for certain patients, dry-needling might be the best strategy as it appears to fill in just as the others, yet without infusing a drug into the body. Different patients report that infusion of lidocaine or potentially a steroid works better for them.

Proof proposes that TPIs can alleviate neck pain for a considerable length of time, weeks, or months in certain patients. In any case, all patients ought to be cautioned that the underlying not many infusions can be very painful. The muscle may really go into a more profound fit before it in the long run unwinds. Patients typically notice an emotional increment in their capacity to move their neck and shoulders after TPIs. The key with TPIs is for the patient to all the while experience active PT to retrain the muscle to remain in a casual state.

Trigger Point Injection
How Botox Works

Most pain specialists suggest an underlying preliminary of week by week TPIs for four to about a month and a half, and afterward reassessment to check whether the patient is encountering a positive result. Once more, recollect it is of most extreme significance that during this TPI preliminary, the patient is likewise taken on an active PT program.
What's happening: Botox for Pain?
In the course of recent years, some pain specialists have been infusing botulinum poison (Botox, Myobloc, Dysport) into trigger points.
How accomplishes that work to mitigate pain? This poison (truly, a similar one used by Hollywood sorts to expel wrinkles!) works by hindering a muscle compound, acetylcholine, which keeps the muscle incapable to contract or go into fit for a while. Different synthetic compounds that may cause pain, inlcuding Substance P, glutamate, and CGRP, may likewise be obstructed by a specific sort of this poison. Despite the fact that this treatment seems to work for certain patients with a more drawn out span of muscle trigger-point unwinding, it's not satisfactory whether it gives favorable circumstances over the more seasoned TPI procedures for all patients. It might be that simply embeddings a needle into the myofascial trigger point (dry-needling) might be similarly effective for some patients.

WARMTH TREATMENT PROVIDES TEMPORARY RELIEF
With the appearance of another kind of warmth wrap (ThermaCare), we have seen numerous promotions touting the use of this sort of treatment for a wide range of pain, including neck pain. In spite of the fact that there is anything but a lot of proof to help heat envelop treatment by the treatment of neck pain, it might give some transitory relief to some neck pain patients without causing any symptoms or dangers.
CRANIOSACRAL THERAPY HAS NO SIDE EFFECTS

A few patients with neck pain acquire significant pain relief and improved capacity with craniosacral discharge treatment and osteopathic control performed via prepared specialists. In spite of the fact that we as nervous system specialists don't comprehend or have faith in the hypothesis of fundamental biowaves and cerebrospinal waves that are at the center of craniosacral treatment, we need to concede we've had a few patients with neck pain report huge profit by craniosacral discharge treatments. What's more, there are no reactions.

REMEDIAL MASSAGE AND ACUPRESSURE WORK FOR SOME
Some proof recommends that helpful back rub and pressure point massage treatment may profit a few patients with neck pain. Likewise with different treatments, such treatments ought to be matched with an active PT/exercise program.

What's going on: Do-It-Yourself Hot Trigger Point Release?

One rising kind of warmth treatment uses a focused warmth source pointed legitimately at the myofascial trigger point. Called central warmth trigger-point (FHTP) treatment, this novel treatment acts simply like a TPI, yet you can do it without anyone's help as opposed to heading off to a specialist's office for treatment. We've had some achievement in treating patients with FHTP, despite the fact that at the hour of this composing no investigations had been led.

Would I be able to purchase a device for this at the drugstore? As of the composition of this book, no device is specifically promoted as a FHTP treatment. Be that as it may, one device, called Zeno, is accessible in certain drugstores and on the web. FDA-affirmed to treat skin inflammation, this device has a focused warmth source and a clock that controls the measure of warmth applied to the skin so as not to cause a consume.

How would I realize where to point the device? It's straightforward. Locate the tight, delicate bunches in your muscles, tendons, and ligaments (see "Examination Findings: Trigger Points in the Neck") and apply the central warmth source with a moderate level of weight on the skin overlying the trigger point.

STRESS MANAGEMENT TECHNIQUES RELAX THE MUSCLES

The stress response has been appeared to cause a compounding of muscle fits in muscles that are causing neck pain. In this manner, it bodes well that stress management strategies, for example, unwinding, symbolism, and biofeedback, can assume a significant job in the treatment of neck pain.

MENTAL TREATMENTS RELIEVE THE MIND AND NECK

Many neck pain patients have depression from the steady, crippling pain they experience. Likewise, numerous patients whose pain started after a mishap, for example, a whiplash injury may have post-horrible stress issue. If you have any of these mental conditions, you should look for mental treatment, as this treatment will assist with diminishing your mental issue, yet additionally your pain.

Treatments to Avoid in Managing Neck Pain

PASSIVE PT WILL NOT WORK

Shockingly, numerous PT programs center around passive, "delicate feely" treatments, for example, delicate back rub, ultrasound, and hot showers. In spite of the fact that these sorts of PT procedures may cause you to feel better incidentally, they won't treat, resolve, or fix your neck issue.

NERVE BLOCKS ARE NOT THE ANSWER

Most pain medication specialists concur that there is no job for nerve obstructs in the treatment of chronic neck pain for most of patients.

SPINAL CORD STIMULATION IS A VERY LAST RESORT

In spite of the fact that there is proof that spinal string incitement might be good for certain patients with different kinds of neck pain, it is our conclusion this ought to be saved as an absolute final retreat for patients with neck pain.

Examination Findings: Trigger Points in the Neck

The neurological examination in patients with neck pain due to myofascial brokenness is totally typical. Nonetheless, clear anomalies are found on direct examination of the muscles of the neck. When the specialist surveys the neck muscles, the person in question will discover myofascial trigger points, tight and delicate muscles that are painful. Frequently, tenderly pushing on trigger points will recreate the entirety of the pains that a neck pain quiet encounters.

SURGERY IS NOT USUALLY THE FIX FOR NECK PAIN

Numerous patients are mistakenly told by their primary care physicians and specialists that their neck pain is caused by a carefully correctable issue, when as a general rule the issue is because of chronic myofascial brokenness. There is positively no job for surgery in the treatment of neck pain related with myofascial pain, the most well-known cause of neck pain. Nonetheless, there are remarkable ailments that cause neck pain where surgery might be justified.

MUSCLE RELAXANTS ARE REALLY SEDATIVES
In spite of the fact that drug organizations have for quite a long time showcased the following drugs as "muscle relaxants," in actuality they don't have any obvious muscle relaxant properties! No drug has been appeared to significantly fix the fit of chronic myofascial conditions. Because these drugs demonstration progressively like Valium, causing significant sedation, we don't suggest them for most patients.
Carisoprodol (Soma)
Baclofen (Lioresal)
Cyclobenzaprine (Flexeril)
Dantrolene (Dantrium)
Metaxalone (Skelaxin)
Methocarbamol (Robaxin)
Orphenadrine (Norflex)
Diagnosing Neck Pain

Radiology tests, for example, X-beams, CT checks, and attractive reverberation imaging (MRI), are frequently ordinary (however recall that many middle-age and more seasoned people have swelling circles in their necks that are not answerable for their neck pain). Electromyography (EMG) might possibly exhibit irregular muscle fits. The consequences of an EMG are regularly totally typical in individuals with neck pain.
Less Common Causes of Neck Pain

Most by far of neck pain is expected to myofascial brokenness in the muscles of the neck and shoulders. In any case, there are less regular causes of neck pain that you ought to know about. We depicted a few of these in part 1 on back pain, for example, spinal stenosis and ankylosing spondylitis, albeit here the issue is in the neck district. Some different less regular causes of neck pain incorporate the following:

CERVICAL SPONDOLYTIC MYELOPATHY

What's going on here?

This condition is likely the most widely recognized cause of spinal string issues in grown-ups more established than fifty-five. With age, degenerative changes happen in numerous segments of the cervical (neck) spine, remembering for the vertebral joints, the intervertebral circles, and the tendons and connective tissue. With these changes, in the long run the spinal line becomes crushed.

Diagnosis:

On neurological examination:

• The quiet gripes of irregular shortcoming and tangible observation in the arms. In extreme cases, the legs may work unusually as the condition advances.

• Muscle squandering (loss of muscle mass) might be obvious in the hand and fingers.

• Abnormal reflexes

• Upon flexing of the neck, the patient may feel an electrical sensation down the back (Lhermitte's sign).

• An MRI or CT examines shows irregular narrowing of the cervical spinal channel.

Symptoms:

• The quiet has a stiff neck.

• Crepitus (grinding, streams, and pops) are felt and heard in the neck with development.

• Weakness; sharp, shooting pains; dull, throbbing sensations; and deadness or shivering in the arms and hands are normal.

• With chronic extreme sickness, shortcoming in the legs and feet and stiffness and awkwardness with strolling happen.

Treatment:

• This is one of the uncommon situations where numerous specialists prescribe early careful treatment to open the cervical trench space.

OSTEOPOROSIS

What's going on here?

Osteoporosis is a chronic condition where the bones become feeble and weak because of loss of bone thickness. This is normal, with at any rate 20 percent of ladies beyond 50 years old having osteoporosis. All bones become frail and can break. When the neck bone (cervical vertebrae) cracks, it can cause chronic neck pain.

Neck Pain Explained

Numerous patients create neck pain following a mishap that brought about a whiplash sort of injury. When a mishap includes your neck, it is the typical capacities of the muscles encompassing your vertebrae (i.e., neck issues that remain to be worked out) stiffen to secure your vertebrae and your valuable cervical spinal rope which is watched by your vertebrae. As a rule following a couple of days or weeks, these muscles step by step lose their stiffness and come back to their ordinary loosened up tone. Be that as it may, for obscure reasons, in certain individuals these muscles stay in a stiff and spastic state, in the long run sinking into a consistent condition of fit, similar to a chronic corked thigh in your neck muscles.

In some cases individuals who work at a PC throughout the day can create neck pain because they are overusing their neck muscles. Your body and neck weren't made to be kept despite everything, gazing at a PC screen for a considerable length of time and hours. In this way, once more, make a point to extend, and if you're feeling sore, enjoy a reprieve and don't overuse those muscles.

CHAPTER FIVE
A BRIEF TOUR OF THE NERVOUS SYSTEM

Comprehend the life structures of how your body makes pain. We realize you need to turn the page (or flick your tablet finger), however don't! The reason for this segment isn't to turn you off, however to turn you on to how your body makes the view of pain. Trust us—it's imperative to find out about your nervous system with the goal that you can all the more likely comprehend your pain, so read on! Here, we will follow your pain signal from its introduction to the world in the peripheral nervous system, into your spinal string, lastly up to your brain.

Peripheral and Central Nervous Systems

The nervous system is subdivided into two sections: the peripheral nervous system and the focal nervous system. The peripheral nervous system comprises of the entirety of the nerves in your skin, muscles, and organs that movement to and from the spinal line. Your spinal string and brain make up your focal nervous system. Basic, right?

Ordinary pain signal's movement

The Role of the Peripheral Nervous System in Pain

To rehash: Your peripheral nervous system comprises of the entirety of the nerves in your skin, muscles, and organs that movement to and from the spinal line. The nerves of the peripheral nervous system are comprised of two fundamental sorts dependent on what they do: your engine nerves and your tactile nerves. The engine nerves go from the spinal string and travel to your muscles. When actuated, these engine nerves cause your muscles to move (by either contracting or expanding the muscle).

Your tactile nerves are a higher priority than the engine nerves concerning pain (no surprise). Tactile nerves, as their name infers, transfer data about different sensations you might be feeling. Tangible nerves are further separated dependent on their size: enormous tactile peripheral nerves and little tangible peripheral nerves.

HUGE NERVES SENSE VIBRATIONS
Have you at any point had a specialist put a tuning fork on your toe or finger? For what reason would the specialist do that? This is the manner by which your primary care physician tests how well your enormous peripheral tangible nerves are working. Enormous peripheral tactile nerves distinguish data about vibrations. To test how your enormous tangible nerves are functioning, a specialist will hit a tuning fork, causing it to vibrate, and afterward place it on your body parts, normally your huge toe, and ask you when you quit feeling it vibrate. Moreover, these enormous nerve filaments are the ones that help you (and your brain) make sense of where your body parts are in space (this is called proprioception). For example, close your eyes and put your hand over your head. If your huge peripheral tactile nerves are working ordinarily, you realized that your hand was over your head without looking. Be that as it may, if these nerves are not working effectively, you would have no clue where your arm was. This can occur in individuals who create neuropathy. Individuals with enormous fiber neuropathy are not ready to tell where their feet are when they are strolling in obscurity, and may therefore feel reeling, causing them to outing or fall.
LITTLE NERVES SENSE PAIN AND TEMPERATURE

Presently how about we get some answers concerning your little tactile nerves, which are increasingly significant when it comes to pain. These nerves will be invigorated, for example, by jabbing the skin with a pin. Little tactile nerve filaments distinguish this incitement and send this painful data from your body to your spinal line. These nerves can likewise recognize temperature data. That is the reason a specialist may here and there put a cold or hot item on your skin, to test how well these little peripheral nerves are working.
Two things can happen when the little tactile nerves are harmed. Once in a while a patient will lose their capacity to feel pain and temperature in the skin territory of that nerve. These individuals

should be cautious because they may hurt themselves without acknowledging they are doing as such. For example, they may consume themselves from burning hot shower water and not feel it. Or on the other hand they can be strolling with a rock in their shoe and not notice it.

In other patients, the inverse can occur. When these little tangible nerves get harmed or excited, they can really get hyperactive and extremely touchy. If this is the situation, little tactile nerves cause pain when there's actually no motivation to feel it. When this occurs, the little tangible nerves cut off, a frayed electrical wire, and continually impart pain signs to the spinal string and brain.

How Your Nerves Talk to Each Other

As you will see, we don't have one major nerve that movements from our skin or muscles as far as possible up to our brain. Numerous nerves are associated en route. These nerves need to converse with each other for data to be passed along starting with one then onto the next. Nerves speak with each other in two significant manners: electrically and synthetically.

ELECTRIC AVENUE

A nerve resembles an electric link, with the electric flow beginning toward one side of the nerve and making a trip to the flip side. The electric link bit of the nerve is known as the axon. When the present beginnings in a single finish of the axon, it will consequently venture out to the flip side.

Be that as it may, when this electric flow arrives at the finish of the principal nerve (we should consider this Nerve A), a basic thing occurs. The accepting (Nerve B) must choose whether this electrical data is deserving of proceeding with the message along its axon, carrying it closer to the brain. In this way, regardless of whether the nerve signal arrives at the space between two associated nerves (called the neural connection) there is no assurance that the signal will consequently move into the following nerve. In the least difficult case, the electric flow itself decides if the signal being referred to is passed along to the following nerve. If there is sufficient electric vitality, the green light is given and the electrical data is basically moved starting with one nerve then onto the next (Nerve A to Nerve B). Notwithstanding, as a rule, another factor will decide if the signal moves along: concoction communication.

Synthetic Substances Modulate Electric Signals

Synthetic substances called synapses adjust electric communication along the nerves. Synapses are delivered in the primary (Nerve A) when the present arrives at the finish of its axon. Nerve A's synapses are then discharged into the space (the neurotransmitter) between Nerve An and Nerve B. Connected to the start of Nerve B (the side confronting the neural connection) are receptors, similar to mitts whose sole reason for existing is to get specific synapses from Nerve A. The system works like a lock and key—when the fitting synapse (the lock) ties to the receptor (the lock) it causes the entryway to open. When the receptor is opened the data from Nerve A is moved to Nerve B.

Neurotransmitter communication

In any case, when Nerve A's neurotransmitter key discovers Nerve B's receptor lock, it doesn't naturally imply that the "entryway will open," allowing data to be passed into Nerve B. A few neurotransmitters will open the lock and pass the signal to Nerve B, a procedure called excitation. Notwithstanding, other neurotransmitters will bolt the entryway much more tightly and prevent the data from being moved into Nerve B, a procedure called restraint.

OK? You may need to peruse this a few times, however once you do, it's truly cool! Presently read on because, as most things in life, it ain't that straightforward. Proceed to the following segment to perceive how things can get much cooler!

The "Pain Gate" in Your Spinal Cord

Along these lines, presently Nerve A's synthetic neurotransmitter key is inside Nerve B's receptor lock. If the neurotransmitter can figure out how to open the receptor, the data will proceed toward the spinal cord. How about we take a gander at the master plan. Recollect the enormous peripheral nerves? They likewise help to move the pain signal along. Both the enormous and little peripheral nerves (from the skin or muscles) combine together onto the spinal cord, Nerve B. In other words, the pain nerve in the spinal cord (Nerve B) gets data from both the enormous (engine and proprioception) peripheral nerves and the little (pain and temperature) peripheral nerves. How do these two kinds of nerves cooperate?

THE GATE CONTROL THEORY

In 1965, to clarify how the pain nerve in the spinal cord (Nerve B) uses the data from both the enormous and little nerves, two pain researcher "divine beings," Patrick Wall and Ronald Melzack, formulated the Gate Control Theory. The Gate Control Theory expresses that, similar to a bygone era scale, Nerve B in the spinal cord gauges the entirety of the data it gets from the enormous and little tactile nerves. The measure of (+) pain data (electrical and concoction) originating from the little nerves is weighed against the (-) pain data (electrical and synthetic) being sent by the huge nerves; in other words, the data from the little peripheral nerves is "excitatory" and the data from the huge peripheral nerves is "inhibitory." The spinal tangible nerve in the spinal cord (Nerve B) is constantly including the entirety of the (+)s and (-)s that it is accepting. The job of the spinal cord nerve is fundamentally that of "gatekeeper": Should it let the pain signal pass or would it be a good idea for it to prevent it from continuing? If you're a Monty Python fan, it resembles the Black Knight in Monty Python and The Holy Grail!

If there are more (+)s than (-)s, the pain data is allowed to go into the spinal cord tactile Nerve B and proceed to the following nerve in the brain. If the (-)s exceed the (+)s, the pain signal is halted and doesn't proceed up the spinal cord to the brain. Bodes well, right? This procedure of including and subtracting pain signals in the spinal cord from the little and enormous nerve strands got known as the Gate Control Theory.

Since 1965, this theory has increased a staggering measure of supporting proof with respect to what befalls the pain signal, and is commonly acknowledged by pain researchers and doctors around the world.

Gate control theory

Your Most Important Organ: The Brain
After the Gate Control Theory turned out to be generally acknowledged, a significant new scientific finding was made: Your brain assumes a significant job in controlling your pain. How you are feeling or your thought process your pain directly affects what befalls the pain signal in the spinal cord, and in this manner hugy affects how much pain you feel!

FROM THE SPINAL CORD TO THE BRAIN AND BACK

Your brain has an immediate connection to Nerve B in your spinal cord. Your brain sends nerves legitimately into a similar pain district of the spinal cord as do your little and huge peripheral nerves. What's more, wouldn't you know it, your brain can likewise send both excitatory (+) pain signals and inhibitory (-) pain signals. The brain then likewise has a vote concerning whether the pain signal will proceed ready or stop in the spinal cord. In other words, your brain balances the entirety of your pain signals even before the pain signals arrive at it. Contribution from your brain can either amplify (increment) the pain signal or hose (decline) the pain signal as it leaves the spinal cord on its way up to the brain. Well that is intriguing!
We will examine this in more profundity later right now. Until further notice, how about we accept that the pain signal has been given the green light at the spinal cord and the pain data has been moved to Nerve B. What occurs straightaway? Once in the spinal cord's Nerve B (called the spinothalamic nerve tract), the pain signal essentially makes a trip up to the brain. The spinal cord goes about as a channel, a straightforward electric link, moving the pain signal from the peripheral nervous system, along the spinothalamic tract, and into the brain.

Once in the brain, the pain signal goes to a region called the thalamus. The thalamus is a structure in the brain that demonstrations like a major city train station. Here, nerve signals originating from all pieces of your body show up to make their first connection in the brain. When the pain signal shows up here, it very well may be coordinated to different brain regions simultaneously, including zones answerable for the sensation, feeling, and recollections related with pain. The signal can likewise be sent to engine regions of the brain, liable for your development reaction to the pain. The brain won't just "see" or sympathize with your pain, yet in addition trigger an activity plan concerning how you ought to react, as to your conduct, your emotions, and your physical developments.

CHAPTER SIX
HOW YOUR BRAIN RESPONDS TO PAIN

To start with, we should find out a little about how the brain functions. Most researchers trust it is the most unpredictable machine at any point made. Surely, without our brain we would not see any pain (really, we were unable to see anything by any means). The sensations and emotions of pain happen because of complex communications among a wide range of parts of the brain.

As we talked about before, after the pain signal goes from the peripheral nervous system through the spinal cord lastly arrives at the brain, the signal spreads quickly to a wide range of districts of the brain. The brain is a heap of interminable systems that are continually conversing with and working with one another. Nobody brain locale can work without anyone else; to work at its most elevated potential, every district should be in steady communication with numerous other regions in the brain.

Pain preparing is no special case. Numerous locales of the brain constantly impart to decide the cause of the pain and the best reaction to the pain you are feeling. When gotten by the brain, the pain signal can take various ways to deliver different reactions. In any case, paying little heed to the specific way, the final product should consistently be a unified, incorporated, and strong reaction. In other words, all the pieces of your brain need to cooperate to shape a reaction that bodes well and encourages you adapt to your present circumstance. (For example, subsequent to being ruined by a lion, you would prefer not to be dreadful and sad and end up running straightforwardly into the lion's mouth!)

How pain functions in the brain

How about we investigate these different exercises and the brain districts that are included.

The Brain and the Sensation of Pain

As we just talked about, when the pain signal arrives at your brain, it goes to a zone called the thalamus. The thalamus lies profound inside the center of your brain and is where a wide range of sorts of sensations, for example, vision, hearing, and smell, all make connections. For the impression of pain, subsequent to visiting the thalamus the pain signal goes to the sensory cortex (the worm-like covering of the brain). The sensory cortex has a wide range of regions, every one devoted to different faculties and body locales.

The sensory cortex is thought to assume significant jobs in the impression of pain. Initially, it decides the pain's power (i.e., the pain signal's quality) and the area of the pain (e.g., arm, leg, or back). The sensory cortex then names the pain as being acceptable (like exercise pain) or awful (as in a potential substantial physical issue). It is significant for your brain to make this qualification with the goal that it realizes what to do straightaway. Would it be advisable for you to cry and pull your hand away (e.g., if your hand is contacting a hot tea kettle), or would it be a good idea for you to overlook the pain and continue focusing on your running (e.g., when you are running a long distance race)? This marking of the pain as fortunate or unfortunate is basic in chronic pain.

The Brain and the Emotion of Pain

As you presently know, pain is constantly connected with a negative passionate reaction, in any event, when you're working out. It shouldn't feel better (except if you're a masochist!). All in all, what some portion of the brain is liable for this enthusiastic reaction? This is an inquiry that keeps on bewildering neuroscientists and rationalists the same. As of now, researchers assume that a locale in the brain called the limbic system might be fundamental for us to encounter both great and awful emotions. Science has additionally appeared, in human brain examine considers, that the pain signal consistently goes to the limbic system. Truth be told, there is proof that in certain kinds of pain, the pain signal can go legitimately from the spinal cord to the limbic system without going through the thalamus. Furthermore, the limbic system, including the amygdala, stores significant recollections, including ones urgent to your endurance—along these lines, you can perceive any reason why connections to the pain signal would be useful.

The Brain's Autonomic Nervous System and Pain

The autonomic nervous system (ANS) is made out of a few structures inside the brain that are additionally essential for endurance. The ANS, similar to the limbic system, is an old piece of the brain (all creatures, regardless of how clever, have this piece of the brain) that controls your blood flow, heartbeat, and breathing rate. The ANS is associated with other brain territories and to other organs in the body, which cooperate to make and execute the stress response—the "battle or flight" response.
Huge numbers of the ANS brain districts are straightforwardly associated with pain and its emotions. These locales incorporate numerous pieces of the limbic system, for example, the foremost cingulate cortex, amygdala, periaqueductal dark, and nerve center. The ANS additionally has connections to the peripheral nerves that go to your skin, muscles, veins, and understudies. You will see further how this brain and body parts cooperate to make the stress response happens consequently.

CHAPTER SEVEN
The Many Benefits of Yoga

Regardless of whether you're unpracticed with yoga, you've presumably heard others discussing it. You may have even heard reports of its numerous advantages. While you may harbor starting wariness about the usefulness of yoga, present day look into is currently accessible to back up a large number of the cases detailed by yoga experts.

In all honesty, numerous famous people depend on yoga! Stars, for example, Jennifer Aniston, Lady Gaga, Adam Levine, and Kate Hudson have acknowledged yoga for helping them get fit as a fiddle for different film jobs. They have likewise used it to help them intellectually center, mend from wounds, and to shield themselves from re-injury. A few big names have even acknowledged yoga for helping them conquer addictions and face unbelievably stressful life challenges.

Yoga is not really a snobby action, so don't give those svelte ladies access charming leotards deceive you. It's an overwhelming type of physical preparing. Numerous expert competitors depend on yoga. LeBron James, Shaquille O'Neal, previous NHL goalkeeper Sean Burke, and Blake Griffin depend on it. "Yoga can be hard." says John Capouya, creator of Real Men Do Yoga. "Not bed-of-nails painful, simply extreme. You're in for a requesting, physically testing exercise here."

Obviously, you don't need to be a VIP or a genius to appreciate the advantages of yoga. Nor do you need an ideal body. While the stars may be able to employ first rate teachers, you can at present appreciate the advantages of yoga any place you are. All you need is this book and the eagerness to educate yourself.

When you genuinely see all the beneficial things yoga can give, all things considered, you will feel much increasingly certain and propelled to give it a shot. It is safe to say that you are thinking about whether yoga merits your time? Take several minutes to familiarize yourself with a portion of its stunning advantages. Yoga:

Advances adaptability. Yoga can step by step slacken your muscles and increment the adaptability in your joints while holding their respectability.

Improves brain work. 20 minutes of yoga can hone your psychological concentration and improve your memory.

Encourages you create solid and adaptable muscles. It prompts assurance from chronic conditions and can lessen the probability of falls and wounds.

Secures against coronary illness. Yoga can lower your danger of heart-related conditions, for example, excessively high or low pulse, dangerous glucose levels, and elevated cholesterol.

Gives you immaculate stance. Poor stance can cause a huge number of joint and muscle issues throughout the years, yet realizing how to adjust your head appropriately over your spine can extraordinarily lessen the measure of strain on your back. Yoga builds your body mindfulness, making it simpler to embrace and continue acts that maintain a strategic distance from over the top stress on any one joint.

Can assist you with coming to and keep up a solid weight. Research has indicated a relationship between's predictable yoga practice and a decline in body weight. Yoga can likewise help the digestion and bolster the progress from fat to muscle tissue.

Shields your joints and ligament from mileage. Yoga includes a full scope of movement, which urges your body to furnish your joints and steady tissues with the supplements they have to stay sound and solid. It can help decrease the pain and stiffness of joint inflammation and diminish the odds of creating other conditions that limit physical development.

Can improve your sexual coexistence. Research has discovered that four months of yoga can expand the sexual exhibition of the two people. It upgrades blood flow to the private parts and strengthens the sphincter muscles, alongside expanding adaptability, quality, mental center, and absolute body mindfulness. To put it plainly, yoga can give a huge lift to your sexual exercises.

Protections your spine. Certain yoga positions can help strengthen your spinal plates, which go about as safeguards for your vertebrae and advance appropriate skeletal arrangement. When your back is appropriately adjusted, it secures your nerves and allows them to convey unreservedly all through your body, giving wellbeing and all-around prosperity.

Assists with recuperating chronic headaches. A few examinations have demonstrated that reliable, long haul yoga practice can assist with settling or lessen the event of chronic headaches. Specialists presently accept certain yoga positions help forestall physical misalignment while assisting with fighting off mental stress, in this way calming headache symptoms and limiting headache triggers.

Upgrades bone wellbeing. Since numerous yoga positions influence your own body weight, yoga is an extraordinary method to strengthen your bones. The act of yoga can likewise advance solid cortisol levels, which enables your issues that remains to be worked out calcium.

Battles off yearnings. The University of Washington reports that yoga positively affects diet mindfulness. The individuals who practice yoga are substantially more aware of the necessities of their bodies and therefore of what they eat and drink. It is simpler to pick sound tidbits when you know about how undesirable bites sway your body.

Lifts your blood course. Yoga builds blood flow by loosening up your muscles. Better blood flow increments cell oxygen levels, which can help all aspects of your body perform all the more effectively.

Moves chronic back pain.

Yoga builds muscle quality and adaptability. This has been demonstrated to facilitate various painful

Lifts your insusceptible system. When you continue a specific yoga position, it assists with flushing out your lymph hubs and invigorate different inner organs. This gives your body a more noteworthy bit of leeway when battling contaminations, tumors, and other infections.

Improves richness. While there are scarcely any examinations that help yoga's certain impact on richness, many accept that by assisting with decreasing stress, yoga adds to expanded fruitfulness levels in ladies.

Helps your heart. Yoga presents are extraordinary for heart wellbeing. The more you hold a specific position, the more your heart will work to supply the vitality your body needs to support the posture. Certain stances, similar to the mountain and the simple posture, open up the heart and its encompassing district to expanded dissemination. The seat, the triangle, and the cobra really require your heart to work more earnestly.

Breathing is too essential to even think about overlooking; yoga's two-to-one breathing proportion, where you breathe out for twice the length you breathe in, has been appeared in a few examinations to improve heart wellbeing even as it helps course.

Paces headache recuperation. Ever lament each one of those beverages you appreciated the prior night? Certain yoga models (for example, the feline dairy animals and the carcass) center on working out your thyroid organ and wringing liquor created poisons from your liver and kidneys. They can likewise support your digestion, which would then be able to work to determine aftereffects in a progressively productive way.

Can diminish circulatory strain. Two British investigations have indicated that, contrasted with dormancy, the carcass really causes a drop in circulatory strain.

Facilitates asthma symptoms. One investigation has indicated that yoga can ease mellow to direct asthma symptoms in grown-ups, because it advances careful breathing systems and incites solid unwinding.

Normal mind-set improvement. A few examinations have demonstrated that rehearsing yoga can build the measure of serotonin in your brain and abatement the measure of cortisol. More elevated levels of serotonin are connected to expanded sentiments of bliss.

Helps people with Multiple Sclerosis. Proof currently shows that yoga may help those with MS by expanding flow, boosting their disposition, and improving their physical capacities.

Can diminish glucose. Studies have connected yoga legitimately to diminished degrees of awful cholesterol and expanded measures of good cholesterol, making it a lot simpler for diabetics to deal with their glucose. The bow, the plow, and particularly the tree, when rehearsed on a customary, expanded premise have helped numerous diabetics to come back to sound glucose numbers.

Yoga tends to the essential driver of glucose spikes: stress. The profound breathing that goes with numerous asanas advances unwinding of body and psyche while the physical positions upgrade appropriate working of systems that direct cortisol and serotonin creation and discharge.

Lifts your memory. Specialists accept that a decrease of mental and physical stress can assist individuals with focusing and organize their considerations in a productive way. Right now. The tree and the lotus both help reliable discernment.

Energizes center. Research shows that reliable commitment in yoga can improve coordination, memory, and response times.

Can postpone signs of maturing. Rehearsing yoga can enable your body to wash down itself of poisons, which can postpone noticeable signs of maturing.

Loosens up your nervous system. Since yoga stances and breathing can cause you to unwind, it can loosen up your nervous system's battle or-flight drive, liberating you to create a quiet, keen reaction to challenges.

Lifts your vitality levels. Steady yoga can reliably help your digestion and lift your vitality levels.

Improves your parity. Yoga is extraordinary for improving your stance, which is an incredible initial step to all the more likely parity. Indeed, even before you find a good pace where you remain on one leg, rehearsing yoga can balance out your parity.

Lessens your body's sodium levels. Yoga can diminish the degrees of sodium in your body in two different ways. To begin with, your muscles use up sodium as they agreement to support a yoga position. Also, numerous yoga asanas empower your kidneys, expanding their capacity to flush overabundance sodium from your body.

Discharges strain. We unknowingly develop strain in muscles without acknowledging it. A prime example happens when a perilous street or thick traffic lead us to hold the guiding wheel firmly as we drive. Continued, this extremely strong grip can prompt chronic strain, irritation, and muscle weakness. Yoga can assist you with getting mindful of which muscles are conveying pressure and can assist you with loosening up them.

When muscles unwind, they channel the development of poisons and increment the course of blood, oxygen, and supplements to the zone's tissues. This, thus, encourages the recuperating of muscle strands, which prompts more grounded muscles that work without lifting a finger.

Expands your red blood cell check. Research has demonstrated that yoga can help support the quantity of red blood cells in your body.

Encourages rest. Research recommends that the loosening up nature of yoga can help energize a superior night's rest. Specific yoga presents are designed to get ready psyche and body for times of rest.

Increments and keeps up deftness skills. Yoga is an extraordinary method to create and keep up excellent deftness; it's considerably more effective than gaming. The body-mindfulness fostered by yoga can likewise expand your profundity observation.

Advances appropriate breathing strategies. Studies recommend that the individuals who practice yoga are less inclined to take enormous swallows of air. Yoga likewise forestalls shallow breathing by including specific guidelines for controlled, full breaths as a major aspect of every yoga exercise. Legitimate breathing lifts dissemination, helps the invulnerable system, energizes unwinding, and invigorates consistent discernment, alongside a large group of other advantages.

Secures your stomach related system. Stress can disturb stomach related problems, for example, ulcers, obstruction, and loose bowels. Yoga can undoubtedly support these conditions. A large number of the yoga presents right now invigorate your absorption. Any of the spinal wind positions are particularly acceptable at helping the stomach related system work easily.

Lifts self-regard. Numerous individuals who take an interest in yoga report feeling an expanded feeling of appreciation and a more prominent capacity to excuse, which thusly gives a tremendous lift to your self-regard.

Can fill in as an enhancement for – or an option to – current medication. Yoga has been used to treat an assortment of conditions for centuries, a long time before the appearance of current clinical modalities. Take constantly your prescription without first counseling your PCP, yet if you can see enhancements in your wellbeing because of rehearsing yoga, don't stop for a second to demand a clinical survey of your condition.

Still not persuaded of the amazingness of yoga? Here are a couple of all the more brisk realities:

Individuals have been rehearsing yoga for at any rate 5,000 years. There are in excess of 100 different yoga represents; their execution can extend from slow and delicate to quick and extraordinary.

Yoga can target pretty much every territory of your body. It can knead interior organs not effortlessly came to by any type of back rub.

Yoga can furnish your body with a finish however low-sway exercise.

Research proposes that yoga can give as quite a bit of a cardiovascular exercise as vigorous exercise.

Yoga can be the ideal non-serious gathering movement.

Yoga is exceptionally reasonable; you can spend alongside nothing to gain proficiency with the essentials. Then again, you can contribute extensive wholes to guarantee you get the best proficient educators, the ideal apparatuses, and effective learning materials.

You can rehearse yoga anyplace – outside on a beautiful radiant day or inside, paying little mind to the weather.

Yoga requires insignificant gear. Numerous individuals use yoga mats to limit slipping, sliding, and awkward sitting on a hard surface, however it's not completely important to possess one. A few people likewise use yoga balls, squares and lashes, however once more, you can exercise effectively without them. A towel can fill in for a lash as a rule, a solid book or metal jars of nourishment can sub for yoga squares, and a cover can fill in as a makeshift yoga tangle.

You can rehearse yoga regardless of whether you have a wellbeing condition. Simply talk about your expectations with your primary care physician already. All through this book I will alert you to contraindications for specific states of being. Certain stances will require adjustments, while other stances ought to be dodged altogether, in view of your physical limitations. Yoga is very conceivable – without a doubt, it can frequently reduce symptoms – for people with coronary illness, hypertension, diabetes, elevated cholesterol, and joint inflammation.

Pre-birth yoga is accessible for ladies who need to remain solid and fit as a fiddle all through pregnancy. A few postures strengthen muscles you will use in the birthing procedure, while others will stimulate you and help you through those early long stretches of lack of sleep after your infant is conceived. There are postures to assist you with awakening and others to assist you with getting ready for rest. Post birth anxiety can be lightened also, since both the breathing practices and numerous yoga presents help to adjust the emotions.

Whether you're in flawless wellbeing or you live with any scope of physical or passionate difficulties, yoga can help improve your personal satisfaction. It can forestall infection, limit symptoms, and can give you unprecedented emotional wellness benefits.

Yoga can straightforwardly improve your general feeling of prosperity, which can assist you with keeping up a positive mind-set and a peppy mentality. Yoga has been found to develop self-acknowledgment just as self-control. It can help reduce threatening vibe and lift social skills.

Above all, yoga is anything but difficult to learn and ace. Specialists prescribe a few days per week from thirty minutes to an hour and a large portion of every, most extreme, as the perfect measure of time to spend rehearsing yoga. Regardless of whether you just go through one hour seven days, aggregate, on yoga, you can in any case experience the entirety of its stunning advantages! So far as that is concerned, even five minutes daily can demonstrate supportive, so if you just have that much time between exercises, use it carefully on yoga. You will love it.

CHAPTER EIGHT
MEDITATION CHALLENGES

Challenge is a monster with a gift in its mouth.
Tame the monster and the gift is yours. — Noela Evans
At this point, you've had the chance to begin to rehearse formal meditation for quite a while and you may have encountered different difficulties en route. This part will survey a portion of the more typical challenges that can emerge.
Expanded mental fretfulness: or on the other hand monkey mind

One normal protest from the individuals who are simply beginning to rehearse meditation is that the very endeavor to move brings about a more prominent anxiety of mind. Once in a while this happens because it is just when you begin to ruminate that you understand how active your mind is. You become mindful of the considerable number of contemplations and sentiments that are ordinarily there, however you've never focused on them, and you may feel that your mind is getting noisier or more disturbed than it at any point was already. Nonetheless, this might be a sign that your mind is getting calmer. You're simply getting mindful of how uproarious and requesting your contemplations and sentiments have consistently been. Undoubtedly your mind was everywhere more often than not. Meditation allows you to see and reduce the measure of prattle your mind takes part in. It prompts a condition of loosened up alertness that can likewise be called thought mindfulness.
As contemplations emerge that have nothing to do with your breath (and this is inescapable), you don't need to blow up or restless with yourself. Recognize that you have lost focus and without making decisions about yourself, delicately return the focus of your consideration regarding your breath. Seeing what diverts you will give you understanding and really makes you a stride nearer to keeping up your focus. Along these lines, when you experience the jabbering of what is known as the monkey mind, the most ideal approach to deal with this circumstance is

essentially to analyze the musings, then let them go, and return your mind to the focus you are taking care of.

Timing

In the most recent week did you contemplate reliably? Or on the other hand was it difficult to make time in your calendar or discover when other individuals would disregard you? Maybe you thought that it was difficult to get into a steady daily schedule. Consider conversing with relatives to get them to collaborate so you can take some continuous opportunity to do your proper meditation. Some of the time relatives see the advantages of day by day meditation in you before you do. If that occurs, a relative may remind you, "Isn't it time for you to do your meditation today?"

A predictable time each day works for certain individuals, particularly if you wind up hitting the hay around evening time having not "got around to doing it." If you tend to nod off during meditation, which is a genuinely basic introductory perception, maybe thinking before anything else may work better for you.

If you are in the workforce, reflecting straight after work on showing up home may work better for you. If you are in a hurry toward the beginning or end of the workday, you can have a go at using your vehicle at noon. Park it somewhere calm, and ponder. Be that as it may, we should underscore this: kindly don't think while driving. Try not to try and consider doing that!

Kids and Pets

Little youngsters and pets are in some cases an issue for meditators, yet a few people find that their pets in the long run start resting discreetly when their proprietor is pondering and doing it as well. Or on the other hand they leave their pets outside the room entryway while meditation is in progress. More established kids now and then join a parent for the meditation.

Reflecting promptly in the first part of the day prior to the more youthful kids wake up, or when they're at school, or when you're sitting tight for them in the vehicle outside their extracurricular exercises are for the most part alternatives you could attempt. We recall the brilliant picture introduced by Saki Santorelli, who took over running the Mindfulness Program at Massachusetts Medical School from Jon KabatZinn. Saki would contemplate each early daytime sitting cross - legged on the floor with a major cover folded over him, into which one of his little kids would once in a while vanish, as though it were a wigwam.

Falling Asleep

Falling asleep is another basic concern. If this is an issue for you, maybe you could take a stab at pondering in a sitting position rather than resting, or during the day rather than at night. If you are as of now restless and meditation is helping you to rest, we state "pull out all the stops" because lack of sleep exacerbates pain and it's harder to adapt. Be that as it may, then it is fitting to include a meditation prior in the day, and check whether you can remain conscious and alert for that.

If you can never remain alert reflecting even while sitting, you despite everything can do all your proper practice as strolling meditation, or as yoga stances, or as mindful development. Falling asleep during meditation may be a safeguard instrument against pain, or a sign of the exceptional lack of sleep that a significant number of our chronic pain patients endure because of their pain or to the side effects of their medications.

Uproarious Environments

From the start, you may find that clamor upsets you, however as you become progressively polished at pondering you may find that you can contemplate through commotion, and even make it part of your meditation experience. In any case, this isn't so likely when you are new to meditation. Pneumatic penetrates outside in the street will justifiably cause difficulty, yet with training even that may get workable for you.

The Hospital Fire Alarm

One day when we were in the third seven day stretch of class, we were ruminating as the alarm began its puncturing screech through the emergency clinic's amplifier system. Not surprisingly, I made note of the way that in a mending organization it appears to be crazy to me to have such a problematic commotion—a different tone without a doubt could be similarly as useful in its ability to alert—and I had a mental image of each emergency clinic patient's resistant system ending in its tracks because of the stress of the clamor.

However, as it began, I noticed that class members to my right had not moved a muscle and those to one side had bounced. The difference was those to my right were graduated class and had been rehearsing meditation for a while and those to one side were "novices."

Abstain from Meditating When You Have Too Much Pain or Too Much Medication

Finding the right time to rehearse formal meditation additionally includes picking when your pain isn't even from a pessimistic standpoint. Keep in mind; you're not doing it to escape pain. Your pain may subside when you ruminate, yet it likewise may not. You may realize that a few hours after a portion of medicine you are in your best pain-controlled time: that might be the best time to settle down for a meditation. Yet, if prescription makes you sluggish or gives you brain haze, it will neutralize the unmistakable mind you can accomplish with meditation, and you may not receive as much in return. For example, high dosages of a portion of the anticonvulsants taken for pain can shield you from capitalizing on the reflective work.

Here and there patients in our training have revealed their minds are more shady than typical because of their medications, and they particularly notice the difference if they can fall off of pain medications subsequent to accomplishing this work. They report getting increasingly out of the meditation and mindfulness when they have a clearer mind. In those conditions, and if you believe you are gaining ground and may make do with less drug, it's surely worth examining with your recommending doctor whether eliminating your prescription slowly would be prudent, so you can capitalize on this work with your mind.

Emotional Stress

The reason for meditation is to "appear" in your own life, and not really to feel better. We live in a culture that has a fear about torment. Commercials everywhere reveal to us how to be glad. All things considered, enduring is viewed as something we should attempt to get away. We're not specific enthusiasts of enduring ourselves but rather we do realize that by focusing on our enduring we can learn numerous valuable exercises. If during meditation practice, you see the enduring as too incredible to hold up under, note it, and proceed onward. Come back to it again later, when you feel more grounded. Be that as it may, don't stay away from it altogether; enduring has a lot to educate us.

On occasion of significant stress in your life, you may not feel persuaded to rehearse meditation and mindfulness, however those occasions are likewise times that very little should be possible to help deal with your pain with prescription. Prescription isn't probably going to fill in also when your stress is extreme, and your rest is of low quality. In this way, on occasion of expanded stress it might feel just as it may not be conceivable to contemplate by any means, particularly if you are unfamiliar to it; in any case, there is another option: development meditation like strolling meditation, yoga, or mindful developments may work the best for you.

Doing combating with back up plans, businesses, and courts can be a horrendous time over-stacked with stress. Nonetheless, when settlements have been come to and you realize what your money related viewpoint is probably going to be, progress can be made. Both mindfulness and pain often become progressively reasonable, and you may even have the option to push ahead and improve.

It's such a lose-lose situation circumstance! When legal advisors inquire as to whether a patient is probably going to show signs of improvement than the person in question is right now, and will the patient ever have the option to join the workforce again, the attorneys would prefer truly not to hear, "Well, when the stress of this case is finished, and this patient realizes what their money related circumstance will be later on, the patient will probably improve; and whether the individual can ever work again is bound to have a constructive answer once this bad dream has finished!" Showing signs of improvement after lawful or protection fights are over isn't malingering. It's exceptionally difficult to have an uplifting attitude about your future and your capacity to restore when you are battling a huge organization for cash to put nourishment on the table and a roof over your head.

Flashbacks and anxiety

We really accept that as often as possible there are past occasions, often as far back as youth, that underlie the powerlessness of the body to recuperate in an opportune manner. If you've had an injury that had an immense effect from quite a while ago, during meditation those recollections may ascend to the surface. All things considered, presently that there are less interruptions, your mind is more clear. If such recollections come to you, they likely should be watched. In any case, you can begin by mindfully "sitting" with recognizing they are there; from the start, maybe under the outside of your mind. Allow them to come into focus step by step more than a few sittings. There's no compelling reason to battle with how to manage painful recollections. Simply sit with them.

If such contemplations and recollections are too alarming, talk about them with your doctor or therapist. As they air pocket to the outside of your mind, they may require some work, which you may or probably won't have the option to do alone. In any case, fight the temptation to stuff them back down into your intuitive mind. This is such a chance to push ahead, past them, because, assuredly, they weren't benefiting you in any way when they were stuck in your intuitive. Such recollections resemble a contamination profound inside a careful injury: we can suture over the top, however an injury never mends appropriately until the disease is cleared out from the bottom up; at exactly that point will it recuperate.

By seeing numerous individuals in our classes experiencing this procedure, we've come to understand that occasionally individuals are more scared of feeling emotional tional pain than they are of physical pain. Truth be told, here and there the physical pain is an interruption from feeling the emotional pain and is simpler to manage; and, tragically, physical pain is an increasingly "authentic" pain to the outside world. All things considered, it's increasingly adequate to tell your boss that you have a headache and need to return home than to state you feel too discouraged to work and need to leave. And, now and then, it appears as though your body knows this and encourages you along by making an interpretation of your emotional distress into the physical pain, for example, of a headache.

Committing to daily meditation

If you live alone, have barely any responsibilities, and have not built up an everyday practice for pondering, do you despite everything find that by sleep time you haven't yet discovered an opportunity to ruminate? It's tragic to state, yet obvious, that the less we need to do, the less we do. This is another type of deconditioning notwithstanding the debilitating of the muscles that you aren't using. If this is so for you, we ask that you watch it as a reality. Try not to bounce on the mind train to misery and depression about it. You should simply locate a reliable time of day to sit officially and focus on a specific timeframe to ruminate.

Presenting a nonstriving attitude

In particular, subsequent to making the dedication, it is then best just to sit with whatever comes up during your meditation and not endeavor to get anyplace with it. Arrangements and progress discover you during your training; not the other route round. For example, you may have seen that occasionally when you wake in the first part of the day, an answer came to you while you dozed. A similar procedure is valid for meditation. Meditation and rest share a few likenesses in what they can accomplish for your mind and body.

CHAPTER NINE
MINDFULNESS AND WEIGHT LOSS

The vast majority have no clue what number of calories are in the normal biscuit purchased at the general store (around 400 calories for an enormous one, which is a great deal if your daily needs are around 1800 calories), or that sugar is the most addictive substance on the planet. A 12-ounce container of soft drink contains around 9 teaspoons (135 calories) of sugar, yet the calorie content wrote about the side of the can is just for 100 milliliters (ml) while the whole can contains 350 ml.

Mindful Habits for Eating Right

Since you're focusing on food by being mindful, you can set aside the effort to peruse the names, understand the caloric substance, and settle on the right decisions. Today, mindfulness courses specifically focused on weight reduction are offered in numerous urban areas.

In such a class you would discover that it takes around twenty minutes to feel full after you begin eating. So a slower increasingly mindful method for eating gives you more noteworthy knowledge into when it's a great opportunity to stop. Cleaning your plate isn't something you should do, presently that you're not sitting during supper with your mother encouraging you to eat everything on your plate. That was then—this is presently.

At your next dinner your new mindfulness may bring about putting less on your plate. Mindfully, you may purchase a littler beverage at the ball game and a little popcorn at the cinema—without the artificial spread. You become mindful of the hankering you may understand in the wake of eating something sweet. If you experience such a hankering, you can go to your breath and trust that the hankering will pass. The day may come, through mindful practice and seeing how addictive sweet foods are, that the remainder of the chocolate mousse can remain in the cooler without coaxing you to wrap it up each time you enter the kitchen.

Your skeleton has been moving you for quite a while yet it ages. It is thankful for any assist you with canning give it, particularly your knees and lower back. Less weight converts into less mileage, which converts into less pain. You may have been on autopilot for a really long time. Right now is an ideal opportunity to be mindful about what and the amount you put into your mouth.

Food and Pain

One of our patients with low-back pain saw that she used to eat a ton of foods containing an artificial sugar and that when she'd disposed of that from her eating routine, her pain diminished. Aspartame, one of the artificial -sweeteners, is likewise usually connected with triggering headache cerebral pains.

Migraines and Food

If you're a headache sufferer, aside from the way that it is typically familial, all things considered, you've just discovered certain foods are headache triggers.

A transport driver who took our course understood that he had been taking a nutty spread and banana sandwich to work each day, without realizing that the two foods were headache triggers. He'd been off labor for a while, and in spite of the fact that he had significant stress in his family, he understood this was in any event a contributing factor to his ceaseless migraines. He came back to work subsequent to finishing the course, ruminates normally, and has remained in the work-power all the more effectively from that point forward.

Headache food triggers incorporate chocolate, citrus organic products, matured cheeses, red wine, and there are numerous others. A trigger is something that can make you increasingly helpless against building up a headache. In any case, it may not cause one unfailingly or just without anyone else. A mix of headache triggers, not really all food triggers, can make you progressively helpless against building up a headache migraine. Lacking rest, dozing late in the first part of the day, or having a stressful week followed by a loose and sans stress end of the week, joined with one of your food triggers, can make you substantially more powerless against building up a headache.

Food, Pain, and Allergy

As you become increasingly mindful of your body and mind's reactions to food, you may discover there are sure foods you truly
can't eat. It may not be as clear as a nut sensitivity, which can
have profound results, or a shellfish or other food hypersensitivity, which may give you rashes, for example, hives. Rather, you
may see stomach pain, swelling, fart, nausea or lethargy subsequent to eating certain foods. Observe: those foods may be sub-
verting you. You simply haven't been giving them your complete
consideration.

Gluten Sensitivity

Celiac infection is an autoimmune illness causing a hypersensitivity to gluten, which is a protein found in grains in a huge range of
foods including breads, cakes, treats, and endlessly. Just a couple
of decades prior, it was believed to be uncommon and influencing
just those who'd first had it in early stages. Today, its rate is believed to associate with 1 in each 100 individuals in the American
populace, and the normal time of beginning is in the forties. It
causes swelling, nausea, and free stool however it likewise can
happen without such clear symptoms. The hypersensitivity to gluten prompts poor ingestion of supplements over all the years the
celiac patient goes undetected.

Similarly as eating a terrible eating routine is a physical stressor
for our bodies and minds, this kind of malabsorption of significant supplements is likewise a stressor and can prompt a wide
range of issues. A portion of those issues are intermittent stomach
pain; osteoporosis, conceivably prompting falling vertebrae; a
more prominent likeli-hood of creating depression and social issues; lymphomas; paleness with its exhaustion and shortcoming;
and, in some cases, a bothersome rash called dermatitis herpeti-
formis. A few people experiencing peevish inside disorder (IBS)
may, indeed, be undiscovered celiacs, and can be screened for it
by a basic blood test called the IgA tissue transglutaminase anti-
body.

James Braly and Ron Hoggan in their book Dangerous Grains
(2002) call attention to that sensitivity to gluten doesn't generally
bring about celiac infection, which can prompt the devastation of
the retaining surface of the little entrail. Indeed, even without
symptoms, sensitivity to gluten can cause the wellbeing dangers
related with it. Braly and Hoggan list numerous wellbeing conditions, including malignant growths, where gluten sensitivity is

overrepresented in that condition's populace, likely was missed in the diagnosis, and likely added to building up that condition. Now and again, the condition was reversible or incredibly improved by expelling gluten from the eating regimen.

One of our patients with Parkinson's sickness, a moderately youngster in his forties, had as of late discovered his shaking was far more regrettable in the wake of eating gluten, and he was at that point killing it from his eating regimen. Tragically, disposing of gluten before a diagnosis can make the blood test appear to be ordinary and can even standardize the intestinal biopsy, which is typically done after a positive blood test affirms the diagnosis. Be that as it may, his perception applies just to him and is of extraordinary incentive to him. Other Parkinson's sufferers may not be gluten-delicate yet he had the option to improve his life by being mindful about what he ate.

It's difficult to eat a sans gluten diet, however it very well may be done and progressed admirably, and numerous items and plans are accessible currently to assist you with disposing of it from your eating regimen. Indeed, even certain eateries and food chains are paying heed by giving decisions and booklets to mention to their customers what their foods contain. You need to get cautious at perusing the marks on the foods you purchase in stores, and to perceive the words that infer shrouded gluten. Whoever felt that licorice contains gluten? Well it does. And soy sauce is matured with wheat, which contains gluten. Sensitivity to gluten is likewise connected with a higher probability of adolescent beginning diabetes, which is additionally an autoimmune condition, and with lactose intolerance.

Lactose Intolerance

Lactose intolerance is considerably more typical since it is perceived as going from gentle to serious, can have a beginning at any age, and can even dispatch in the wake of being extreme during outset. Mindfully noticing that swelling and nausea happen subsequent to eating oat with customary milk, may piece of information you into perceiving that you have this condition yourself. All things considered, if standard milk in tea or cream in a difficult situation, you may understand you have a mellow lactose intolerance. So mindfully you may make your own diagnosis and decide how firmly you respond. If your intolerance to lactose is serious in any case, there are heaps of medications that contain lactose as filler: be careful!

Food, Moods, and Behaviors

We've just talked about the connection between feeling more pain when you are in an irate mood. In her book Food, Teens and Behavior (1983), Barbara Reed, Ph.D., a post trial supervisor, expounded on the transaction among diet and conduct. She discovered that a significant number of the teenagers whom she administered waiting on the post trial process had been eating awful weight control plans at the time they carried out their violations. They ate eats less carbs stacked with trans fats, which have no genuine healthy benefit. Indeed, even some sound foods like milk had triggered abnormal behaviors in specific people, who plainly had quirky responses to those foods. She put these adolescent offenders on solid weight control plans, which they needed to consent to keep up as a state of their probation. Then she kicked back and viewed the adolescents' improved behaviors change them into model residents.

Since we have quite a lot more data about gluten sensitivity, we think it is conceivable that a portion of these teenagers may have been undiscovered celiacs.

Jaimie Oliver, the superstar British culinary expert, probably thought about food affecting conduct when he crusaded to change the substance of school snacks in Britain, as appeared in his narrative TV arrangement. Discovered that his own kids shouldn't endure at the hands of the educational system when they began school, he took on retraining the "supper women" who prepared the profoundly handled foods for their particular youthful customers' snacks. He had a significant fight—because the kids opposed—however cooking great food without any preparation made additional work for the supper women.

School spending plans didn't generally take care of the expense of nutritious foods, and the nonattendance of dietary data among guardians all conspired against him. In the long run, his constancy paid off and British school lunch charge is continuously changing. The capacity of the kids to focus after lunch is climbing, and in one TV scene, an educator, who typically gave asthma inhalers to asthmatic kids at noon, detailed that inhaler use had been definitely reduced: indeed, great sustenance even influences lung work.

The UK is as of now presenting mandatory cooking exercises in schools for kids matured eleven to fourteen to figure out how to cook nutritious foods without any preparation. And beginning in 2008, Quebec has banned French fries, soft drink, and low quality nourishment from candy machines and cafeterias in its schools. These administration activities recognize the job food plays in impacting youngsters' fixation capacities; also they battle stoutness.

The Glycemic Index
We as a whole realize that sugary foods can transform a few kids into a lack of ability to concentrate consistently scatter carbon copies. The glycemic index , which alludes to how quickly each kind of food causes an ascent in blood sugar subsequent to being eaten, is likely affecting everything here. Foods with a high glycemic index are those that cause a quick ascent in blood sugar, which then falls similarly as quickly about an hour in the wake of eating. These limits in blood sugar levels happen because insulin is created in too extraordinary a quantity by the pancreas attempting to react rapidly to drive the sugar into the cells and out of the bloodstream, where elevated levels are perilous.

If you've at any point seen a diabetic in the ER with low blood sugar, you've seen what that does to mood. The individual is forceful to the point of ruining for a battle not long before dropping. Give such people squeezed orange while they can in any case swallow, and they return to being your closest companion! To a less radical degree that transpires too, and is particularly risky if you are inclined to migraines.

Our headache patients on opiates for their pain realize that if we see them in the coffee shop purchasing an enormous coffee with sugar and Danish, they ought to expect war in the coffee shop. If they must be on opiates for migraines, they need to do the better than average thing and eat appropriately!

A precipitous fall in your blood sugar level is downright terrible for you from multiple points of view. When in the low-blood sugar stage, you may feel anxious and argumentive; your capacity to focus is poor; and you're bound to start a quarrel. None of this is useful for any painful condition you may have. The quick ascent of too much insulin causes your body to store progressively fat.

Too much insulin causes you to emit a greater amount of the stress hormone, cortisol, which is likely why you feel nervous.

Joining a food that raises blood sugar level, for example, a grain, with foods that cause a much slower ascend in blood sugar, for example, almonds, allows the insulin discharged by your pancreas to be discharged all the more slowly too. This, thus, slows up the blood sugar ascend from the high glycemic food. So for break-quick, if you consolidated a high glycemic food, for example, grain, with low glycemic foods, for example, nuts and seeds, you'd probably discover you're not all that hungry in the late morning and you'd have a superior mood and more prominent capacity to move later in the day.
Have you seen that you're tenser subsequent to eating certain foods or in the wake of taking certain medications or drinking stimulated beverages? By rehearsing mindfulness you may find that you are increasingly mindful that a portion of your moods impact whether you feel pretty much pain at those occasions. Eating steadily is a central point in stacking the chances so your body and mind work better, which will make it simpler to adapt to your pain.

Mindfulness and Caffeine

The normal chronic pain quiet is restless. You might be attempt-ing to make up for daytime lethargy by drinking too a lot of cof-fee. Multiple cups a day is probably going to cause jumpiness and meddle with your evening time rest. It's normal to know about nine or ten cups of coffee being devoured so as to improve day-time alertness. Increasingly restorative rest is really the best treatment for being alert.
Slow reduction of your coffee admission, regardless of whether you have been devouring it for the most part in the first part of the day, is one approach to oversee poor rest. Note that an abrupt end or a radical drop in coffee utilization can cause disrupting anxiety, much the same as pulling back from some other drug. Af-ter your utilization has been incredibly reduced, others may not perceive the enhanced you. Your non-verbal communication might be a great deal looser after your rest has improved. And recollect, rest is additionally useful for your resistant system,

which should be fit as a fiddle to help the harmed painful pieces of your body, regardless of whether the harm took place years prior.

Fluids and Pain

Not drinking enough liquid, particularly in blistering weather, builds the impression of pain in chronic pain sufferers. The incidental liter of liquid administered by IV restores our patients' pain control without turning to expanding their pain prescription sometimes. This has happened even without the clinical signs of parchedness (loss of skin versatility, lacking pee); nevertheless, deficient liquid causing the whole body to be too dry is a physical stressor for them. Insufficient fluids likewise fuels the obstruction such huge numbers of our patients experience the ill effects of their pain medications.

For example, a few shots of morphine didn't get Gillian, our patient with an ineffectively working entrail, back in pain control for the few hours she was in the ER. Her tongue was so dry it was adhering to the roof of her mouth. After she was given a liter of liquid, she rose from her gurney and went to a Bar Mitzvah that night.

Foods and the Immune System

We are blockaded daily with advertisements for solid foods and now supermarkets are making them substantially more accessible. So we have less excuse for not feeding our bodies with sound foods. Antioxidants, found in numerous foods, for example, apples, blueberries, guavas, dark tea, and dull chocolate, are great for your immune system. A few investigations have connected them with improved proficiency and carefulness of the immune system to prepare for malignant growths (Knight 2000).

Omega-3, a sort of unsaturated fat, which has been demonstrated to be an anti-inflammatory, is significant in giving the structure squares to the membranes of your cells. And numerous investigations have demonstrated the gainful effects of a vegetable-rich eating regimen on lowering the frequency of colon malignant growth.

Vitamins and Pain

Vitamins are additionally significant for individuals with chronic pain. A few examinations have shown the advantages of 400 mg daily of nutrient B2 (Riboflavin) to forestall headache cerebral pains. Of late, nutrient D has been getting a great deal of press because in nations that have cold winter seasons, the individuals are so lacking right now. Supplementation with nutrient D has in some cases reduced pain astoundingly, and not because it helps with forestalling osteoporosis. Besides, a connection has as of late been found between nutrient D insufficiency and higher narcotic portions.

Dr. Michael Hooten, clinical director and anesthesiologist at Mayo Comprehensive Pain Rehabilitation Center, Rochester, Minnesota, detailed at the American Society of Anesthesiologists' yearly gathering in 2007, that in excess of 25 percent of a chronic pain populace going to a pain recovery focus were insufficient in nutrient D. That gathering was on double the normal narcotic portion, and announced less fortunate wellbeing and more awful physical working compared to those on narcotics who were not insufficient in nutrient D.

Exercise

The conspicuous advantages of exercise for mitigating pain barely need conversation; nonetheless, as a pain sufferer, you are bound to ask us, by what means can you exercise? Particularly because you hurt significantly more when you do exercise. Tragically, the painkillers or anesthetic strategies that hinder your pain in some cases veil too huge numbers of pain's notice signs—and cause you to try too hard. Then you pay for practicing with crippling pain. So you land back on the lounge chair for quite a while.

Finding the right parity of exercise to go with medications and clinical systems isn't easy. You need simply enough pain relief to allow you greater development yet less that you'll disregard any admonitions from your body while working out. It is difficult however it very well may be finished.

Indeed, even headache sufferers profit by being in better state of being. They report that when they keep up a normal exercise system they have less migraines and those they do have are less nosy. Showing signs of improvement state of being is additionally prone to expand your versatility to emotional stressors, which might be the reason headache sufferers report less migraines when they routinely exercise. And there's heaps of -evidence for exercise improving results in the management of low-back pain.

Exercise is the one sure treatment to restrain the seriousness of fibromyalgia's effects. It assists with reducing body stiffness and look after portability, which can be an impasse circumstance for the individuals who have serious fibromyalgia, because it causes stiffness and loss of versatility. However, using muscles expands their blood flow and therefore their temperature—so they feel less stiff and are more averse to fit—and using muscles builds their quality. Then the joints these muscles support become less painful.

Practicing likewise expands endorphins, which are the regular inward pain-executioners answerable for sprinter's high. It doesn't need to mean doing anything too truly lively: strolling or swimming is fine.

Since you are getting progressively mindful, you are bound to know when you have arrived at your breaking point and stop. And bound to acknowledge that limit without lament. Making infant strides from the start can incorporate doing the mindful development meditation. If you can oversee delicate Hatha yoga, that would be a great beginning.

Yoga

There are numerous kinds of yoga yet Hatha yoga is the sort portrayed by Jon Kabat-Zinn in Full Catastrophe Living (1991). He remembers its training as a meditation for his mindfulness - based stress reduction program, which he created in 1979, and which has now spread all through the world. Elizabeth Gilbert, in her engaging top of the line book Eat, Pray, Love (2006), clarifies that yoga in Sanskrit is interpreted as association, which means a relationship between the body and the mind. She likewise alludes to the numerous reasons for yoga, including releasing up muscles and ligaments so as to set up the body to keep up yoga positions while reflecting for extensive stretches. It is additionally conceivable to get to otherworldliness through meditation.

In beautiful composition she says: "Yoga is about self-authority and the committed exertion to pull your consideration away from your unending agonizing over the past and your nonstop stressing over the future so you can look for, rather, a position of everlasting nearness from which you may respect yourself and your environmental factors with balance". This is actually what mindfulness encourages you to do. And by moving your body through yoga stances, you can delicately recover the capacity to move once more, definitely more than you might suspect conceivable as of now.

Sleep

Information about the elements of sleep is detonating and sleep laboratories are seeing expanding quantities of referrals. Their referrals are ordinarily over-weight individuals who wheeze and have a high probability of not getting enough oxygen around evening time. The dangerous neck periphery in a male is seventeen inches: over that, a man likely needs to have a sleep study done.

Sleep apnea is a condition where the sleeper stops relaxing for a brief timeframe while asleep. It is described by poor oxygenation around evening time, and has been connected to a higher probability of coronary illness. However, cerebral pains and daytime weakness because of poor sleep are issues too. At our center, we're progressively alluding chronic pain sufferers to sleep labs for study because such a large number of report battling with sleep issues like daytime exhaustion, eager legs in bed, wheezing, and upsetting their accomplices.

Expanding overweight patients' narcotic portions puts them in danger, and even underweight or ordinary weight patients on narcotics have given some sleep apnea issues. Sleep apnea is treated with a cover or nasal prongs connected to a positive aviation routes pressure (CPAP) machine, which conveys a surge of air around evening time, so unhindered breathing can proceed if the body neglects to breath profoundly enough while sleeping. We've likewise observed outrageous cerebral pains and a forceful diabetic neuropathy (nerve damage) pain start a couple of years before sleep apnea was analyzed, and we've wondered if the apnea prompted the seriousness and inability of these conditions.

Sleep Stages

There are five stages of sleep: stages 1 to 4 and quick eye development or REM sleep. A grown-up's typical evening time sleep cycles through these stages about at regular intervals. Stages 1 and 2 are light sleep: it's easy to arouse the sleeper in those stages. Stages 3 and 4 are more profound, slow-wave sleep and rousing the sleeper from those stages is more earnestly to do and the sleeper might be disorientated on waking. It is imagined that the immune system fixes the body from the mileage of the day in the more profound sleep stages.

REM sleep is more connected with dreaming than the other stages are, and we as a whole need a specific measure of REM to be sound. Truth be told, having no REM or too much REM sleep is related with depression. Antidepressants can change the measure of REM sleep the individual taking such prescription encounters. In their book Sleep and Pain (2007), Gilles Lavigne and his col-classes talk about the expanding number of research concentrates in the relationship among sleep and pain. They make it a lot more clear why the body is so poor at working and fixing damaged parts when sleep is deficient long or profundity.

Fibromyalgia patients don't appear to have a lot, if any, slow-wave action sleep in their sleep examines, and here and there these patients review they were poor sleepers in their pre-fibromyalgia days. Some fibromyalgia sufferers display wave structures called alpha interruptions on their sleep analysis printouts, which makes it seem as though they wake up a few times each night. Along these lines, the absence of slow-wave sleep or the interruption of attentiveness is in all likelihood associated with these patients' irritated throbbing muscles and chronic weakness.
If you report you are experiencing difficulty sleeping to your medicinal services supplier, there are moves you can make to improve your sleep: these activities are often called sleep hygiene. They ought to be examined before you have a go at taking sleeping pills or heading off to a sleep center.
Mindfully Observing Sleep Hygiene
Great sleep hygiene tends to the propensities and conditions required for guaranteeing a long and profound enough sleep to advance great wellbeing.
Routine sleep times. It's ideal to attempt to target hitting the sack at the equivalent or comparable time each night. Your body has a stress-hormone diurnal beat that follows the twenty-four-hour cycle of day and night. This stress hormone, cortisol, ought to be at its most elevated level toward the beginning of the day when you need to be alert, and lowest around 12 PM when you need to be asleep. This is associated with the light/dull cycle of our ancestors who had no entrance to the artificial light we underestimate. (It's conceivable these ancestors would be advised to working diurnal rhythms than we do.) Shift laborers and voyagers experiencing plane slack concur that changing sleep times is stressful: to such

an extent that you may feel sick for a few days in the wake of changing work shifts or coming back from a nation midway or more around the globe.

Note that if you're recouping from an illness or you are going away from malignancy, it doesn't bode well to stack the chances against your immune system by coming back to a stressful shift-changing daily practice busy working.

It's likewise essential to attempt to ascend at the equivalent or comparable occasions every morning, in any event, when you didn't get a decent night's sleep. You may be bound to improve sleep the following night than if you sleep late toward the beginning of the day to make up for the lost sleep around evening time.

Eating and drinking. Eating an overwhelming supper near sleep time isn't prudent: it's probably going to keep you conscious. Drinking fluids too near sleep time is additionally an issue if you're probably going to find a good pace night to pee and you experience difficulty falling back asleep. This is likewise risky if you take sleep prescription, which makes you shaky on ascending during the night.

Charged beverages ought to be maintained a strategic distance from near sleep time. For certain individuals, they ought to be maintained a strategic distance from after twelve early afternoons. For poor sleepers, it's prescribed to drink close to two cups of juiced coffee daily, ideally before evening. We've seen individuals gotten totally changed after they've tapered off too numerous cups of coffee daily, and then experienced improved sleep and reduced eagerness. Note that wine and other mixed drinks can likewise keep you wakeful. And when alert around evening time, you may note you long for something sweet to help your serotonin, which is low around evening time: It is easy to gain weight if you have a sleeping disorder.

Cool room. Your body was designed to lower your temperature to some degree during the night when you have substantially less muscle movement. Despite the fact that it's imperative to remain warm, it's additionally critical to breathe cool air. So keep a window open if that should be possible.

Exercise. Practicing prior in the day rather than not long before sleep time upgrades sleep. As expressed over, this may represent a portion of the advantage that exercise gives on the pain of fibromyalgia, because a sleep insufficiency is a central point in keeping up pain and weakness.

Television and/or PC use. Sitting in front of the TV or seeing PC screens has the effect of fooling your brain into believing it's light. So if you experience issues sleeping, abstain from doing this not long before sleep time. Viewing stressful TV programs, for example, murder riddles is additionally prone to keep you wakeful.

Use your bedroom just for sleep and sex. Have you set up your bedroom to be your office, understanding room, and work-out station? Then your mind won't partner the bedroom with serene exercises. It is ideal to keep the bedroom only for sleep and sex. If you should peruse before resting, it's prudent to do that in another room, away from the bedroom, and to pick mitigating understanding material.

Maintain a strategic distance from daytime rests. You might not have rested soundly the prior night yet it might be smarter to expand the time you think rather than rest during the day, which may meddle with the following night's sleep. For the individuals who don't have a sleeping issue, power rests of close to thirty minutes' term are acceptable, however that is altogether different. When you can't sleep, find a workable pace. It's better not to toss and turn or lie there turning out to be increasingly disappointed, yet to find a good pace, room, and accomplish something non-stressful in a repressed light for around ten minutes before coming back to bed. This is when meditation, either sitting still or strolling, can be extremely useful in reducing the gab of your mind, which will allow you to give up, and will remind you not to endeavor to nod off. The more you endeavor to sleep, the less you will succeed. Ruminating and stressing are great sleep deprivers. Mindfulness and meditation truly can assist with reducing these propensities.

Medications. Sleep medications may assist you with finding a workable pace so you can stop agonizing over the absence of sleep. If you would then be able to take it from that point without expecting to keep taking the sleep drugs, that can be useful. In any case, if taken each night, they ordinarily lose their effectiveness after only half a month. And if you attempt to stop taking them, you will in all probability experience bounce back attentiveness, which sends you right back to taking them once more; despite the fact that they don't work well overall.

Slowly decreasing sleep drugs can assist with maintaining a strategic distance from that bounce back, yet know that there are no medications we are aware of, including the calming antidepressants and anticonvulsants, that truly increment the restorative sleep stages, the sleep you need. In addition, a few medications may even keep you wakeful: Individuals shift in their responsiveness. Narcotic medications may reduce the slow-wave further sleep, the very sleep you requirement for mending your body.

Physical stressors

You may have thought of stress as being fundamentally emotional, however indeed, as should be obvious from perusing this part, stressors incorporate physical stresses, for example, and less than stellar eating routine, too much or too little action, poor sleep, and environmental weather and temperature changes. Aside from the weather, if your physical stressors are out of equalization and you become increasingly mindful of them, change will probably happen more than a while to years essentially through your mindfulness—and it will improve how you handle the emotional stressors you experience, as your life unfurls. If you feel much improved, that is as of now far to getting stronger to stress.

The individuals in your life can keep you well and expand your life or they can make you extremely debilitated and abbreviate your life range. Knowing this and getting mindful of your responses to others can make way for improving. Reducing your stressful sentiments can support your mending and reduce your pain.

CONCLUSION

Spinal cord stimulation, otherwise known as SCS, uses electrical stimulation to give pain relief of the back, neck, legs, and arms. It is accepted that electrical motivations will restrain pain sensations from being gotten by the brain. SCS candidates incorporate patients who are experiencing chronic pain and for whom traditionalist treatments have fizzled or possibly careful treatment has not given substantial relief.

Before having a last implant set with a spinal cord stimulator, the patient should experience arrangement of a preliminary implant first. The doctor will sanitize and numb the territory of the back under concern and an epidural needle is put. When the epidural needle has arrived at the spinal channel, a catheter is set through the needle.

The patient isn't totally anesthetized for this preliminary implant method. The explanation is that the doctor needs to solicit the patient so, all things considered from position the patient accomplishes sufficient pain relief of the zone experiencing chronic pain. When the catheter is in the situation for easing pain best an outer force supply and software engineer is appended which supplies power and will allow the patient to wear it for 5 to 7 days. During the week that the preliminary implant is put, the patient will keep a diary specifying precisely how much pain relief is accomplished from the preliminary. If the implant accomplishes satisfactory pain relief, (for example, over half), the patient may proceed onward to a last implant. In any case, the preliminary implant is evacuated in the office at about seven days' time.

The lasting implant is set under sedation and often times general anesthesia. Through a little cut in the lower back, the specialist will play out a little laminectomy or laminotomy, which implies a tad of bone overlying the epidural space is expelled. By then the oar lead can be put into the epidural space and situated properly in the middle for pain relief.

The new oar leads contain more than 10 diodes and there are a lot of projects accessible for pain relief. By doing this, the patient will have a lot of alternatives where to acquire relief from their chronic pain. A fluoroscopic machine is used so as to ensure that the SCS paddle is put suitably, which shows the metallic diodes in fitting position.

When the oar is in the proper position, the generator is then put in the subcutaneous tissue at the top of the buttock district. One needs to verify that it isn't put in a territory the patient will be perched on. The more current generators are excellent in that they allow for reviving outside the skin while the patient is sleeping. The patient is instructed how to shift starting with one program then onto the next for ideal relief.

Does it appear to be astounding that we can achieve tremendous jumps in medication and science yet presently can't seem to make an imprint in eradicating chronic, regular medical problems?

Finding the fix to the regular virus appears to be much the same as finding the lost city of Atlantis!

As clinical natural customers will come to me from all pieces of the wellbeing range: from genuine chronic malady, to weight issues and low vitality. What has surprised me is what numbers of individuals make them thing in like manner: chronic pain.

It is upsetting to perceive how individuals have gotten so accustomed to having the pain, it is an acknowledged consistent in their lives. And as opposed to searching for the answer for disposing of it, they look for management alternatives: drug, exercise, therapy, chiropractors, and the like.

These alternatives all have their place in the recuperating range - indeed, even prescription (briefly).

Be that as it may, shouldn't something be said about disposing of the pain for good? Have we gotten so used to hearing "no" from doctors, other patients, our families, and the media that we accept that is the appropriate response without bothering to pose the inquiry?

For anybody that has had any involvement in the objective setting, self-help, self-awareness mindset - you realize that no doubt about it "take the plunge!" to make a decent attempt, that nothing is unthinkable.

Be that as it may, when it goes to your wellbeing, particularly with a condition that is said to be "chronic" - you surrender. You acknowledge what you're told and the cutoff points you're given.

If pain management is the main choice your doctor gives you, you resign yourself to its long haul nearness in your life.

Is that all there is? In no way, shape or form.

The issue with tolerating restrictions and putting together your recuperation and mending with respect to the encounters of other individuals is it cuts off you to what is really conceivable. It resembles keeping your food decisions to the main section of a menu that is 16 pages in length.

So what's the initial step, the most significant pivotal advance to evacuating and totally discharging a condition like chronic pain for good?

It's relinquishing the conviction that other individuals can characterize your constraints.

That is it.

Connections, family, vocation, wellness, wellbeing, recuperating, health, cash - whatever it is, your restrictions are what you conclude they are.

Do you refuse to set any confine for yourself whatsoever? Go to the leader of the class, because now nothing is distant.

The customers I see share another thing practically speaking besides chronic pain - they are happy to make that progression, they don't acknowledge "management". They need answers, they are open (regardless of whether it's only a smidgen) to the chance of being without pain.

And with that specific expectation, we can discover their answers and an outline is framed for recuperating and discharging the pain for good.

Numerous individuals are experiencing peacefully chronic back pain and stress over not ready to discover a fix. Home pain relief and elective treatment can help in numerous occurrences, particularly for the individuals who are looking for lower back pain relief. It has been accounted for that just in the United States of America alone; there is a normal 31 million individuals with lower back pain at some random time.

If you ask the elective specialists, a significant number of them feel that back throb can be lowered by as much as 60% if you use the right exercises or therapies. Such treatments may speak to individuals looking for non-obtrusive treatments as they would prefer not to turn to medical procedures or ingesting medications like neurontin for chronic pain.

Here are a portion of the regular treatments to calm back pain:

- **Chiropractic:** A qualified chiropractor can analyze the pain and treat it. Clinical investigations have demonstrated that chiropractic care is sheltered and effective. The treatment includes spinal control, prescription, exercise and rest. Be that as it may, not all individuals are reasonable for such treatment, particularly those with history of spinal surgery, experiencing osteoporosis or nerve damage.

- **Acupuncture:** Acupuncture is an elective treatment for pain created by the Chinese numerous hundreds of years back. It includes embeddings sterile needles into specific pieces of the body to give chronic pain relief. Acupuncture has been seen useful when the pain is as too chronic for other treatments to be used.

- **Massage methods**: For years, the craft of back rub has been received as a tool of relief and unwinding. Many accept that back rub can truly help in postural pressure, muscle weakness and word related stress and strain. When executed accurately, rub low back pain can loosen up the muscles to give you the relief and keep the pain from returning. Back rub are milder than osteopathy and chiropractic however they don't comprehend a portion of the basic back issues.

- **Physical therapy and exercise:** There are exercises that you can gain from your physiotherapist to do at home to assuage chronic pain. For whatever length of time that it isn't awkward for you, you can begin them when you can move. This is probably going to be inside the following 1-2 days from the beginning of the assault. Notwithstanding if the exercises disturb the pain, you should stop right away.

The best home back pain relief is as yet taking great consideration of your back in your ordinary exercises. You should exercise often. Try not to slump or droop back when situated and don't hunch when driving, perusing or dealing with the PC. You should take standard breaks by moving around. Never twist your back to lift an overwhelming item.

As a safety measure, consistently look for a doctor's recommendation before you take up any home back pain relief or normal pain treatment, particularly if your pain isn't because of a straightforward physical cause.

The basic facts about chronic back pain relief:

Alongside migraine, back pain is the most across the board neurological grievance in the United States. Any pain that endures for longer than 90 days is considered to be a chronic condition. Chronic pain is every now and again dynamic, and deciding its cause is often difficult. The danger of lower back pain because of spinal degeneration or circle malady increments with age.

Generally low back pain is treatable without surgery. Drug is much of the time effective in treating intense and chronic pain. This may include a mix of over-the-counter and physician recommended drugs. Check with a doctor before consuming medications for continuous chronic back pain relief, as specific medications, much over the counter, are perilous during pregnancy, may cause tiredness and other side effects, may struggle with other prescriptions, and can even prompt liver damage.

Anti-inflammatory pain relievers, sold over the counter, incorporate headache medicine, ibuprofen, and naproxen. These may reduce growing and stiffness, just as irritation, and often ease mellow to direct low back pain.

Anticonvulsants, mostly used in treating seizures, might be of advantage in treating some nerve pain and might be endorsed alongside analgesics.

Counter-aggravation scouring creams or splashes influence the skin's nerve endings to supply sentiments of cold or warmth, and to dull pain signals. In like manner, topical analgesics can diminish irritation and animate blood flow. Often, these mixes contain salicylates, an ingredient used in oral pain prescriptions that contain headache medicine.

Certain antidepressants have exhibited pain relief, autonomous of their effect on mood, and can help with sleep. Such medications change brain science levels to dull vibe of pain, and to lift mood. Some more current antidepressants, for example, SSRIs, are under examination for pain relief effectiveness.

Medicine narcotics, for example, hydrocodone, oxycodone, codeine, and morphine are used to give chronic pain relief, just as extreme instances of intense pain, however just for a brief timeframe and under doctor supervision because of their serious side effects and habit potential. A few experts are even persuaded that chronic use of such drugs is unsafe to the back pain sufferer, as they can expand depression and even increment pain.

Spinal control includes manual modification of spinal structures by authorized pros, for example, chiropractors, using exercises and influence to restore portability.

If back pain doesn't improve by means of the above regular techniques, patients may wish to ponder the following options for further research: acupuncture, biofeedback, interventional therapies running from neighborhood infusions of anesthetics, steroids, or opiates into influenced zones. Chronic steroid infusion use may bring about mischief to a person's working.

Where there is proof of vertebrae cracks, for example, those caused by osteoporosis, a few methodologies incorporate footing, TENS, ultrasound, and different other outpatient treatments. A portion of these procedures, once stylish, are currently disapproved of by numerous experts. The best methodology, in any case, is the one that works for you, and the most ideal approach to find out about your alternatives is to do your own examination, and pose a lot of inquiries.

If all else fails, surgery may give relief from chronic back pain. In any case, recuperation is slow, and lasting loss of adaptability is conceivable. As back surgery is an obtrusive methodology, and not constantly fruitful, it is just educated in cases concerning peripheral nerve damage or dynamic neurological ailment.